The International Library of Bioethics

Volume 107

The *International Library of Bioethics* comprises international and interdisciplinary volumes on foundational and applied issues in bioethics. The series focuses on perennial topics of aging, mental health, preventive medicine, medical research issues, end of life, biolaw, and other areas of bioethics, whilst expanding into other current and future questions involving the living world. The *International Library of Bioethics* examines the role of bioethics against the background of increasing globalization and interdependency of the world's cultures and government.

The series explores meaningful ways to answer the questions of how to direct biotechnology to human and other living things' ends, how to deal with changed values in the areas of religion, society, and culture, and how to formulate a new way of thinking. That is, to create a new, practical bioethics.

The international Library of Bioethics welcomes book proposals representing the broad interest of the series' focus. We especially encourage proposals addressing aspects of changes in biological and medical research and clinical health care, health policy, medical and biotechnology, and other applied ethical areas involving living things, with an emphasis on those interventions and alterations that force us to re-examine foundational issues.

Natasha H. Williams

Artificial Intelligence and Healthcare

The Impact of Algorithmic Bias on Health Disparities

Springer

Natasha H. Williams
School of Law
Loyola University Chicago
Chicago, IL, USA

ISSN 2662-9186 ISSN 2662-9194 (electronic)
The International Library of Bioethics
ISBN 978-3-031-48261-8 ISBN 978-3-031-48262-5 (eBook)
https://doi.org/10.1007/978-3-031-48262-5

This Springer imprint is published by the registered company Springer Nature Switzerland AG
The registered company address is: Gewerbestrasse 11, 6330 Cham, Switzerland

Paper in this product is recyclable.

For my parents, Frank and Helen Williams

Acknowledgements

I would like to thank my daughter, Ashley, for her love and support. I would also like to thank all who inspired and encouraged me.

Contents

Chapter 1
Artificial Intelligence and Algorithmic Bias

Abstract Medical advances such as telemedicine, precision medicine, genomics, and artificial intelligence (AI) have revolutionized the practice of medicine and the treatment of disease. These technologies, especially AI, promise to advance the quality of patient care, lower health care costs, improve patient treatment outcomes, and decrease patient mortality. To achieve these ambitious goals, AI depends upon massive streams of data from various sources. Section 1.1 defines AI. Section 1.2 describes data. Section 1.3 explores data and algorithmic bias. Section 1.4 discusses race-based algorithms. Section 1.5 summarizes key points in the chapter.

Keywords Artificial intelligence · Algorithmic bias · Machine learning · Data quality · Training data · Race-norming

1.1 Artificial Intelligence in Health Care

Imagine a 54-year-old male visits his family doctor because he has a few nagging health issues. He has diabetes and sees his doctor regularly but thinks his symptoms may be unrelated to his diabetes. He has a cough that rattles his chest, swelling in his legs, loss of appetite, and modest weight loss. He has health insurance, so he is not concerned about paying for his medical care. Based on his symptoms, the doctor orders laboratory tests to identify the possible cause of his ailments. Since the patient has diabetes, the weight loss could be attributed to his diet and may require an insulin adjustment. The doctor waits for the lab test results before making any significant changes. He thinks the likely culprit is a severe chest cold and prescribes an antibiotic, telling the patient to go home and get some rest. A few weeks later, the patient feels better. His test results did not flag anything out of the norm. The leg swelling has ceased, his appetite has increased, and his weight has remained steady.

Two months later, the patient sees blood in his urine. He returns to his doctor, and after another series of tests, the doctor determines that it is a urinary tract infection. The patient is scheduled for same-day surgery to insert a stent in the infected area to drain it. He is also prescribed antibiotic therapy. After the surgery, the patient recovers

N. H. Williams, *Artificial Intelligence and Healthcare*, The International Library of Bioethics 107, https://doi.org/10.1007/978-3-031-48262-5_1

and resumes his usual daily activities. One day, the patient notices that his vision is blurry. He thinks it is related to his diabetes. Knowing that the disease can cause vision changes, he thinks he might need new glasses. He goes to the ophthalmologist who sees something very abnormal. He tells the patient that he has tumors in his eyes. Immediately, the patient goes back to his family doctor and is admitted to the hospital for a series of tests. This time the diagnosis is dire. The patient has cancer throughout his entire body, affecting his lungs, liver, bones, brain stem, and eyes. After several months of specialist consultations, exploratory biopsies to determine the primary cancer source, chemotherapy, and radiation, the patient dies within five months of diagnosis. The primary type of cancer is never identified. The year is 1996.

Over twenty-five years later, medical technological advances such as telemedicine, precision medicine, genomics, and artificial intelligence (AI) have revolutionized the practice of medicine and the treatment of disease. These technologies, especially AI, promise to advance the quality of patient care, lower health care costs, improve patient treatment outcomes, and decrease patient mortality (Krittanawong et al. 2017). To achieve these lofty goals, AI depends upon massive streams of data from various sources. Some of these data sources are medical records, electronic health records, clinical trial data, and scientific journals. For the cancer patient from 1996, the diagnostic capability of AI may have been an additional tool in the doctor's toolbox to assist in diagnosing and treating his disease. AI in health care is still in its infancy, so it may not have saved his life. Nevertheless, it may have improved quality of life. Despite the potential of AI in health care, the patient still may not have benefited from its diagnostic and treatment capabilities because he was an African American male. Often, racial and ethnic minority groups are underrepresented in data. The lack of data inclusivity may build an inherent bias into training data, and ultimately AI systems. Training data are used to train, or teach, algorithms. Therefore, as AI moves forward, many racial and ethnic minority groups may be left behind. The impact of AI on health disparities has been largely understudied (Williams 2019).

Medicine has evolved from mysticism and superstition to the science that created a vaccine to protect society from the modern-day plague of SARS-CoV-2, the virus that causes COVID-19 disease (Kaba and Sooriakumaran 2007). Likewise, AI has evolved incrementally, building upon the successes and failures of the scientists that laid its foundations (McCorduck 2018; Nilsson 2010). In 1950, Alan Turing, a British mathematician and logician, wrote the paper, *Computing Machinery and Intelligence*, which introduced the Turing Test (McCorduck 2018; Nilsson 2010). It proposed that a machine was considered to have the ability to think like a human if it could mimic or imitate human actions. The "imitation game" became the equivalent of AI holy grail (McCorduck 2018). The term "artificial intelligence" was first coined in 1956 by John McCarthy, an assistant professor of mathematics at Dartmouth College in Hanover, New Hampshire (McCorduck 2018; Moor 2006; Nilsson 2010). In 1955, McCarthy and his colleagues[1] submitted a proposal to the Rockefeller Foundation

[1] McCarthy was the lead writer. The other colleagues were Nathaniel Rochester, IBM Corporation; Claude E. Shannon, Bell Telephone Laboratories; and Marvin L. Minsky, Harvard University.

to organize a workshop to study how to create machines that can simulate human learning and could think like humans (Moor 2006). This six-week workshop, the Dartmouth Summer Research Project on Artificial Intelligence, was held in 1956 (McCorduck 2018; Moor 2006; Nilsson 2010). This pivotal event is considered the birth of the research field of artificial intelligence (McCorduck 2018). Today, AI decision support tools aid in hospital discharge planning, identify the patient risk of hospitalization or readmission to the hospital, monitor signs of sepsis, and predict patient deaths (Robbins and Brodwin 2020). In the prediction and treatment of disease multiple sclerosis (Eshaghi et al. 2021), colorectal cancer (Augustus and Ellis 2018), and breast cancer (Himes et al. 2016).

The definition of AI is varied and broad. Some describe it as the ability to systematically solve complex problems or a logical agent that will achieve the best expected outcome (National Science and Technology Council, Committee on Technology 2016; Scherer 2016). The common underpinnings are to create machines that "automate or replicate intelligent behavior," improve upon human performance, or think like human beings (National Science and Technology Council, Committee on Technology 2016, p. 7; Domingos 2015). Table 1.1 that defines terms that are key to understanding AI.

It is within these constructs that AI is categorized into three different types. These are narrow artificial intelligence or weak AI, artificial general intelligence or strong AI, and artificial superintelligence or super AI (Naudé and Dimitri 2019). Narrow AI detects patterns in a dataset to make predictive models. Narrow AI is task oriented. Examples of narrow AI include games, virtual assistants, self-driving cars, image recognition, document review systems, content recommendation, and language translation (Matheny et al. 2019). On the other hand, general AI is analogous to human intelligence. It can teach itself and obtain human consciousness (Russell and Norvig 2010). This type of AI does not currently exist (Livingston and Risse 2019; National Science and Technology Council, Committee on Technology 2016). Artificial superintelligence occurs when AI surpasses human intelligence. Needless to say, that type of AI does not exist either (Naudé and Dimitri 2019).

As computers become increasingly powerful and the fields of computer science, data science, engineering, and neuroscience advance, AI will continue to mature, evolving from its current state to what it aspires to become. One constant is that AI tools, especially machine learning models, need data for their training and to make their predictions or to perform tasks. Therefore, it is important that data are diverse, representative, and free of bias.

1.2 What Are Data?

Data are everywhere. They are generated by global position systems (GPS), online shopping, movie streaming, surfing the internet, sending a tweet, posting a picture, using smart thermostat sensors, and the list goes on. Definitions of big data range from the technical to the general. In the simplest terms, big data are massive complex

Table 1.1 Terms used in artificial intelligence

Term	Definition
Artificial intelligence	A branch of computer science that studies "enabling computer systems to perform tasks normally requiring human intelligence" (U.S. Department of Health and Human Services 2023)
Machining learning	The use of algorithms that are able to "learn by extracting patterns from a large body of data. This contrasts to traditional rule-based algorithms" (IT Modernization Centers of Excellence n.d.)
Supervised learning	"Uses of labeled datasets to train algorithms to classify data or predict outcomes accurately" (IT Modernization Centers of Excellence n.d.)
Unsupervised learning	"Uses unlabeled data. From that data, it discovers patterns that help solve clustering or association problems" (IT Modernization Centers of Excellence n.d.)
Reinforcement learning	"Behavioral machine learning model that is similar to supervised learning, but the algorithm isn't trained using sample data. This model learns as it goes by using trial and error. A sequence of successful outcomes will be reinforced to develop the best recommendation for a given problem" (IT Modernization Centers of Excellence n.d.)
Narrow artificial intelligence	"Task-specific AI" (IT Modernization Centers of Excellence n.d.)
Artificial general intelligence	"Refers to AI that achieves general human-level intelligence … At this point not technically possible" (IT Modernization Centers of Excellence n.d.)
Generative AI	"Generative AI systems create text, images, audio, video, and other content … These systems are trained to recognize patterns and relationships in massive datasets and can quickly generate content from this data when prompted by a user" (U.S. Government Accountability Office 2023)
Training dataset	"A training dataset is used to teach models to yield the desired output and includes inputs and outputs that are correctly categorized or "labeled," which allow the model to learn over time" (IT Modernization Centers of Excellence n.d.)

aggregated streams of data that are difficult to analyze with traditional data processing methods (Hansen et al. 2014). Instead, predictive analytic methods, such as algorithms, are used to identify patterns in the data (Maddalena et al. 2020; Hansen et al. 2014). Algorithms are the instructions to solve a mathematical problem and the foundational building blocks of AI (Broussard 2018). They comb through large datasets to identify patterns and probabilities in the data (Broussard 2018; Livingston and Risse 2019; Naudé and Dimitri 2019).

> Algorithms generate categories for filtering information, operate on data, look for patterns and relationships, or generally assist in analyzing information. The steps taken by an algorithm are informed by the author's knowledge, motives, biases, and desired outcomes. The output of an algorithm may not reveal any of those elements, nor may it reveal the probability of a mistaken outcome, arbitrary choice, or the degree of uncertainty in the judgment it produces. So-called "learning algorithms" which underpin everything from recommendation engines to content filters evolve with the datasets that run through them, assigning

> different weights to each variable. The final computer-generated product or decision—used for everything from predicting behavior to denying opportunity—can mask prejudices while maintaining a patina of scientific objectivity. (Executive Office of the President 2014, p. 14)

Big data have been defined in terms of volume (i.e., data magnitude), velocity (i.e., rate and speed data are generated and analyzed), and variety (i.e., different types of structured and unstructured data) (Maddalena et al. 2020; Gandomi and Haider 2015; Zhang et al. 2017). Some definitions also include veracity (i.e., accuracy and reliability) and value (i.e., obtaining meaningful information) (Maddalena et al. 2020; Gandomi and Haider 2015; Zhang et al. 2017). Other definitions include exhaustivity, extensionality, and complexity as big data elements (Maddalena et al. 2020; Gandomi and Haider 2015). Data are also structured, unstructured, and semi-structured. Structured data consist of numbers and values that are organized into rows or columns, have a predefined framework, consistent format, and offer the ability to query and manipulate (Gandomi and Haider 2015). Examples are an Excel file or database (Gandomi and Haider 2015). Conversely, unstructured data are unorganized non-formatted data that do not have a predefined framework and are difficult to query (Gandomi and Haider 2015). Examples include email, web pages, video, audio, social media posts, and sensor data. Semi-structured data fall in between the two forms. These data do not have a table or database structure, but they contain markers and tags (Gandomi and Haider 2015).

Algorithms are integrated into every aspect of society, including social media, shopping, policing, advertising, employment, financing, housing, and insurance (O'Neil 2016). Not only have algorithms crept into everyday life, but they are also pervasive in nearly every industry, including manufacturing, business, law, education, entertainment, the arts, sports, and health care (O'Neil 2016). In health care, data sources include medical records, administrative records, electronic health records, peer-reviewed articles, clinical trials, wearable devices, clinical registries, insurance claims data, medical imaging, biobanks, laboratory tests, and genomic sequencing data, to name a few (Maddalena et al. 2020; Hansen et al. 2014; Zhang et al. 2017).

Algorithms are used in disease prevention and identification, treatment therapies, and health care administration and management. For example, algorithms identify diabetic retinopathy (U.S. Food and Drug Administration 2018), predict chronic asthma in children (Bose et al. 2021), detect cancerous colon polyps (U.S. Food and Drug Administration 2021), and determine the health care management needs of patients (Obermeyer et al. 2019). High-quality bias-free data are essential to train algorithms to make accurate predictions. Algorithms are only as accurate as the data they are trained with. For example, algorithms have been used in dermatology to distinguish between benign and malignant moles (Adamson and Smith 2018). However, if darker-skinned individuals are not included in the training dataset or they represent a small part of dataset, the algorithm cannot accurately predict skin cancer in this group (Adamson and Smith 2018). Consequently, these predictions may exacerbate health disparities because darker-skinned people are overlooked and do not benefit from the early disease detection that the algorithm provides (Adamson and Smith 2018).

Challenges may arise when medical data are collected for one purpose but used for another purpose, like research (Peek et al. 2014). Data from medical records collected for patient care, which include patient demographics, laboratory tests, clinical notes, physician observations, disease history, medications, treatment history, and clinical therapies, may not provide the necessary information for secondary use in research (Peek et al. 2014). Moreover, critical data may be missing, inaccurate, or mislabeled (Peek et al. 2014). One of the risks of big data is that if the data are not carefully curated and standardized, it will be of poor quality, resulting in inaccurate output (Van Poucke et al. 2015). Therefore, the collection of high-quality data is often a challenge. Data quality (DQ) and data quality concerns are:

> The capability of data to be used effectively, economically and rapidly to inform and evaluate decisions. Necessarily, DQ is multidimensional, going beyond record-level accuracy to include such factors as accessibility, relevance, timeliness, metadata, documentation, user capabilities, and expectations, cost, and context-specific domain knowledge. Data quality concerns are problems of large-scale machine and human generation of data, the assembly of large data sets, data anomalies, and organizational influences on data characteristics such as accuracy, timeliness, and cost. (Karr et al. 2002, p. 2)

The elements of data quality may differ according to the framework used, but some core elements are accuracy, timeliness, and completeness (Karr et al. 2002). In addition to these core elements, data should also be trustworthy. To be trustworthy, data must be applicable, consistent, and reliable to make accurate inferences and predictions (The National Coordination Office for Networking and Information Technology Research and Development (NITRD/NCO) 2016).

1.3 Data and Algorithmic Bias

Bias can occur at multiple levels, from creating and selecting the data itself to the person who is programming and curating the data (Campolo et al. 2017). Bias occurs when the algorithm is trained on data that are not diverse or it measures the wrong outcome variable (Obermeyer et al. 2019). Biased algorithmic outcomes occur in criminal sentencing, advertising, employment, credit qualifications, and same-day delivery service (Datta et al. 2015; Ingold and Soper 2016; O'Neil 2016). For example, Angwin et al. (2016) analyzed a risk assessment algorithm used to assess if a criminal defendant would likely re-offend and found that Blacks were more likely to be incorrectly considered to have a higher recidivism risk than Whites (Angwin et al. 2016; Larson et al. 2016). The data used by the assessment tool did not include race; however, there were other data or proxy variables that could be associated with race (Angwin et al. 2016; Dressel and Farid 2018; Mehrabi et al. 2021).

Algorithmic bias may begin with the data to train the algorithmic model, but it is magnified when the algorithmic tool is deployed and implemented, leading to algorithmic discrimination (The White House and Office of Science and Technology Policy 2022). Algorithmic discrimination occurs when "automated systems contribute to unjustified different treatment or impacts disfavoring people based on their race, color, ethnicity, sex (including pregnancy, childbirth, and related medical conditions, gender identity, intersex status, and sexual orientation), religion, age, national origin, disability, veteran status, genetic information, or any other classification protected by law" (The White House and Office of Science and Technology Policy 2022). It is difficult to root out algorithmic data bias because algorithms are intellectual property, and their decision-making processes are unknown (Broussard 2018; O'Neil 2016).

> ...... there are inherent challenges in trying to understand, predict, and explain the behavior of advanced AI systems, due to the complexity of the systems and the large volume of data they use. The difficulty of understanding machine learning results is at odds with the common misconception that complex algorithms always do what their designers choose to have them do, and therefore that bias will creep into an algorithm if and only if its developers themselves suffer from conscious or unconscious bias. It is certainly true that a technology developer who wants to produce a biased algorithm can do so, and that unconscious bias may cause practitioners to apply insufficient effort to preventing bias. In practice, however, unbiased developers with the best intentions can inadvertently produce systems with biased results, because even the developers of an AI system may not understand it well enough to prevent unintended outcomes. (National Science and Technology Council, Committee on Technology 2016, p. 3)

We do know that if the data are biased, those biases are inputted into the algorithmic model (Broussard 2018; O'Neil 2016). The algorithms themselves may not be inherently biased, but the data training sets they learn from may be. In those scenarios, the biased algorithmic outcome is a function of the biased data. There are many sources of data bias including measurement bias, aggregation bias, and sampling bias (Mehrabi et al. 2021; O'Reilly-Shah et al. 2020). Other types of bias include bias from (1) programmer values and perceptions; (2) historical data that ignore the cultural and stereotypical assumptions embedded in the data and populations that were historically precluded; (3) the lack of data diversity and representation; and (4) data that are race-neutral on their face but biased in their application. Data are subject to these biases, and they can be embedded in the algorithms (Broussard 2018; O'Neil 2016).

1.3.1 Programmer Values and Perceptions

Bias may be introduced through programmer values and perceptions. The datasets are labeled by human beings in supervised machine learning and therefore are susceptible to human biases and assumptions (Campolo et al. 2017). These human biases may originate from unconscious stereotypical beliefs and attitudes, overt bigotry, unawareness, or the lack of context. Furthermore, algorithms are trained on these datasets. For example, a photography application identified Blacks as gorillas (Guynn 2015). Moreover, Buolamwini and Gebru (2018) found that some facial recognition algorithms misclassified darker-skinned women. Some of these errors may be rooted in training data that lacked a broad representation of people, the designer developed an algorithm that distinguishes facial features in some races more than others, or the algorithm designer may have depended upon his own experience in distinguishing facial features (Buolamwini and Gebru 2018; Garvie and Frankle 2016).

Additionally, data bias can result from the type of people in the technology field who develop algorithms, programs, and label data. The lack of women and racial and ethnic minorities in the technology field may create bias because their ideas, perceptions, and values are not represented in these AI systems (Campolo et al. 2017). Some of the reasons for the lack of diversity and representation in the technology field include implicit bias, similar-to-me bias (i.e., preference to hire individuals who are similar to themselves), and the failure to diversify the Science, Technology, Engineering, and Math (STEM) educational pipeline in the United States (U.S.) (Campolo et al. 2017). For instance, the number of degrees awarded to racial and ethnic minority groups in Science and Engineering (S&E) lags critically behind Whites (National Science Foundation 2022). In 2019, the number of S&E bachelor's degrees earned by Whites was 58.8%, whereas only 16.3% of Hispanics, 11.3% of Asians, 8.7% of Blacks, 0.4% of American Indians or Alaska Natives, and 0.2% of Native Hawaiians and Other Pacific Islanders received S&E bachelor's degrees (National Science Foundation 2022). Moreover, the disparity in S&E master's degree recipients was similar: 61.2% Whites, 12.2% Hispanics, 11.3% Blacks, 11.1% Asians, 0.4% American Indians or Alaska Natives, 0.2% Native Hawaiians and Other Pacific Islanders. The same disparities existed for S&E doctoral degrees (National Science Foundation 2022). Whites earned 69.1% of S&E doctoral degrees, and only 10.6% of Asians, 8.4% of Hispanics, 8.1% of Blacks, 0.4% of American Indians or Alaska Natives, and 0.2% Native Hawaiians and Other Pacific Islanders received S&E doctoral degrees (National Science Foundation 2022).

1.3.2 Historical Data Bias

In other cases of data bias, bias in historical data used in training sets may reflect stereotypical assumptions or populations that were historically precluded, which will lead to future bias (Williams et al. 2018). For example, in 2015, a large technology company found that its recruitment tool under development was not gender neutral. The algorithm was trained on 10-year-old data that reflected the technology industry, which at the time was predominately White and male (Dastin 2018).

1.3.3 Lack of Data Diversity and Representation

Data bias occurs when data are not sufficiently diverse to reflect the population because certain populations are not included in the data (Bass and Huet 2017; Knight 2017). For example, in 2022, African Americans and Hispanics or Latinos comprised approximately 13.6% and 19.1% of the U.S. population, respectively (U.S. Census

Bureau 2023). However, it is estimated that only five percent of African Americans and one percent of Hispanics or Latinos are clinical trial participants nationally (The Society for Women's Health Research and the U.S. Food and Drug Administration Office of Women's Health 2011; Vickers and Fouad 2014). This disparity has important implications because racial and ethnic minority groups and socioeconomically disadvantaged populations disproportionately have adverse health outcomes compared to the general population (Zhang et al. 2017). Therefore, it is imperative that their data are reflected in clinical trials.

Clinical trials are research studies performed to evaluate the efficacy and safety of a drug, treatment, medical device, or protocol. Historically, clinical trial data were skewed towards White men, not women or racial and ethnic minorities (Campolo et al. 2017). To identify sex, gender, and racial and ethnic differences and to determine treatment effectiveness and efficacy, the inclusion of women and racial and ethnic minorities is crucial (U.S. Department of Health and Human Services. National Institutes of Health 2017). Unfortunately, clinical trial data can lack adequate numbers of racial and ethnic minority groups and low socioeconomic populations (Branson et al. 2007). Furthermore, the underrepresentation of these groups fails to consider the impact of environmental exposures, stressors, and life experiences that would not be otherwise understood, and these are important considerations for the studies (Branson et al. 2007; Zhang et al. 2017). The inability to recognize these differences may impact clinical trial results, leading to ineffective treatments or interventions that work for only a portion of the population (Branson et al. 2007). Equally important, these research studies generate data. When certain populations, such as women, racial and ethnic minorities, and sexual and gender minorities, are not adequately represented or missing from the data, the efficacy, safety, and generalizability of research results to the larger population are limited (Zhang et al. 2017). To improve data inclusiveness, it is important to include standardized demographic information and social determinants of health in clinical data (Zhang et al. 2017).

In 2009, researchers analyzed the genome-wide association study (GWAS). The GWAS is "an approach used in genetics research to associate specific genetic variations with particular diseases. The method involves scanning the genomes from many different people and looking for genetic markers that can be used to predict the presence of a disease. Once such genetic markers are identified, they can be used to understand how genes contribute to the disease and develop better prevention and treatment strategies" (U.S. Department of Health and Human Services. National Human Genome Research Institute 2021). The researchers found that 96% of the GWAS participants were of European descent (Bustamante et al. 2011; Need and Goldstein 2009; Popejoy and Fullerton 2016). In 2016, Popejoy and Fullerton updated that GWAS analysis and discovered an improvement in the inclusion of individuals who were not of European descent (Popejoy and Fullerton 2016). Nevertheless, the inclusion of individuals of African and Latin American ancestry, Hispanic, and indigenous people improved very little (Popejoy and Fullerton 2016).

Data bias that impacts algorithmic outcomes occurs when certain data are not collected or included in databases or the algorithmic data training sets. Data must also capture the social determinants of health, genetic information, environmental exposures, and health care delivery and outcomes (Zhang et al. 2017).

1.3.4 Race Neutral Data and Bias

Data may be race neutral. That is, race may not be included as a factor in the data analysis. However, even though race is not included, there may be bias in its application because it fails to recognize the institutional, cultural, and socioeconomic factors that may impact the data training set. For example, "an algorithm used to allocate access to disease management support programs was found to include prior use of health care services as a surrogate for disease severity. This led to stark racial disparities in program use because previous use of resources (i.e., health care utilization) itself was indicative of barriers to care and existing health care inequity, thus not accurately representative of need for services" (U.S. Department of Health and Human Services. Agency for Healthcare Research and Quality 2021, 2023). Specifically, Obermeyer et al. (2019) discovered that an algorithm adopted nationwide by health systems to predict whether patients would need additional care management resources identified that White patients would need more care than Black patients, severely underestimating the health needs of Black patients. Once corrected, Black patients receiving additional resources would increase from 17.7% to 46.5% (Obermeyer et al. 2019). When approached by the researchers, the algorithm's developers independently replicated the analysis on its national database of nearly 3.7 million patients, finding that Blacks had almost 49,000 more active chronic diseases than Whites (Obermeyer et al. 2019). When the researchers changed the variable label by creating a variable that combined health prediction with cost prediction rather than using future cost, the bias was reduced by 84% (Obermeyer et al. 2019). The initial algorithm used health care cost data as a proxy for health (Obermeyer et al. 2019). The algorithm was not intentionally racially biased because race was excluded (Obermeyer et al. 2019). However, the algorithm developers failed to realize that Blacks utilized the health care system less than Whites for various reasons, including lack of insurance and access to medical care (Obermeyer et al. 2019). The researchers deduced that the culprit was the data, specifically the label used to measure illness initially (Obermeyer et al. 2019).

1.4 Race-Based Algorithms

Race is a social construct, not a biological or genetic trait. Throughout medical history, race has been used to classify, marginalize, and dehumanize racial and ethnic minorities (Washington 2006). Also, it has been a tool to assert biological and intellectual superiority over these groups (Cerdeña Jessica et al. 2020). In the name of research, race has been an excuse to conduct inhumane experiments that exploit vulnerable populations (Washington 2006). "Race and ethnicity are often used as input variables and influence clinical decision-making and patient outcomes. Because race and ethnicity are socially constructed, their inclusion as variables within health care algorithms may lead to unknown or unwanted effects, including the potential for exacerbation and/or perpetuation of health and health care disparities" (Cerdeña Jessica et al. 2020; U.S. Department of Health and Human Services. Agency for Healthcare Research and Quality 2023; Vyas et al. 2020). Race and ethnicity are often included "by citing observational studies or post-hoc analyses of trial data that demonstrate differences in characteristics or outcomes among different racial/ethnic groups. These studies may be small and unrepresentative, serve to reinforce misconceptions, or assign race/ethnicity as a contributing cause when other factors may be causative, confounding, or modifying the effects of race" (U.S. Department of Health and Human Services. Agency for Healthcare Research and Quality 2023).

In the New England Journal of Medicine article titled *Hidden in Plain Sight—Reconsidering the Use of Race Correction in Clinical Algorithms*, the authors posit that race-based algorithms may perpetuate disparities because they direct additional resources to White patients and not racial and ethnic minorities (Vyas et al. 2020). A partial list of race-based algorithms was identified in the article. These algorithms are routinely used in cardiology, nephrology, obstetrics, urology, oncology, endocrinology, and pulmonology (Vyas et al. 2020).

For example, the Breast Cancer Surveillance Consortium Risk Calculator provides a five-to-ten-year risk estimation of women developing breast cancer (Vyas et al. 2020). The coefficients rank race/ethnicity in descending order of risk starting with Whites, followed by the other race/ethnicity categories (Vyas et al. 2020). As a result, there is a lower risk estimation for anyone who is nonwhite (Vyas et al. 2020). Additionally, the pulmonary function tests use spirometers to measure lung volume and diagnose respiratory disease (Lujan and DiCarlo 2018). In the United States, spirometers use a race correction for Blacks and Asians that erroneously estimates lung function in those groups (Lujan and DiCarlo 2018). Spirometers have a storied history that dates back to the slavery era when it was believed that there were physiological differences between the lungs of Blacks and Whites (Lujan and DiCarlo 2018). The popular idea was that forced labor was beneficial to Blacks because it invigorated their blood (Braun 2015; Lujan and DiCarlo 2018). This racial bias was embedded into the race correction. Moreover, the Osteoporosis Risk SCORE (Simple Calculated Osteoporosis Risk Estimation) captures race as Black or non-Black and assigns five additional points if the person is non-Black (Vyas et al. 2020). The maximum score is 50, which represents the highest risk. This results in lowering the estimated risk of osteoporosis in Black patients, which may delay additional testing, diagnosis, and treatment (Vyas et al. 2020). Furthermore, the Vaginal Birth After Cesarean (VBAC) Risk Calculator predicts the probability of a successful vaginal birth after previously having a cesarean section (Vyas et al. 2019, 2020). The factors inputted into the algorithmic model are age, body mass index, prior vaginal delivery, a prior VBAC, the reoccurring indication for cesarean section, African American race, and Hispanic ethnicity (Vyas et al. 2019, 2020). Because the race correction decreases the estimated success rate for those identified as Black or Hispanic, the VBAC score predicts a lower chance of a successful vaginal birth after a prior cesarean for Black or Hispanic women (Vyas et al. 2019, 2020). The risks associated with cesarean delivery are infection, hemorrhage, and blot clots (Mayo Clinic 2021). Grobman et al. (2021) derived a model that excluded race and ethnicity from calculating the probability of a successful vaginal birth after cesarean (Grobman et al. 2021; Palmer 2021). The updated model performed at the similar level of accuracy as the previous model that included race (Grobman et al. 2021; Palmer 2021). However, it still needs to be validated externally (Palmer 2021).

1.4.1 Race and the Glomerular Filtration Rate (eGFR) Index

In the United States, it is estimated that 35.5 million people have chronic kidney disease (CKD) (U.S. Department of Health and Human Services, Centers for Disease Control and Prevention 2023). Chronic kidney disease occurs more in women (14%) than men (12%) (U.S. Department of Health and Human Services, Centers for Disease Control and Prevention 2023). Approximately, 20% of Black adults, 14% Asian adults, 14% of Hispanic adults, and 12% of White adults have CKD (U.S. Department of Health and Human Services, Centers for Disease Control and Prevention 2023). Risk factors for CKD include hypertension, diabetes, heart disease, obesity, older age, and family history (U.S. Department of Health and Human Services, Centers for Disease Control and Prevention 2023). The estimated glomerular filtration rate (eGFR) is widely used in the United States to measure kidney function. Creatinine, a muscle protein, is a marker for kidney disease and is measured in the eGFR. Since 1976, the eGFR considers several factors: the patient's age, sex, body size, and African American race. However, race is only defined as Black or other (Smith and Spodak 2021). The higher the score, the better the kidney functioning. The debate of whether to use race in the eGFR equation rests on whether (1) it will reduce disparities because early identification will provide patients early access to care and specialty treatment; or (2) its removal may increase disparities because it will no longer capture race, which is an important factor in eGFR (Smith and Spodak 2021).

In eGFR equation validation studies, Black adults had higher creatinine levels when compared to White adults (Vyas et al. 2020; Delgado et al. 2021). The inclusion of race results in Blacks being scored higher, thus presenting with better kidney function, which may not be accurate (Vyas et al. 2020; Delgado et al. 2021). Salman et al. (2021) examined Black patients with CKD and the impact of a race multiplier (correction factor) in the equation to estimate kidney function (Salman et al. 2021). They found that if the race multiplier was removed from the equation, up to one in three of the 2,225 Black patients (33.4%) would be classified to a more severe stage of CKD (Salman et al. 2021). Additionally, almost one in four of the 687 Black patients (24.3%) would be reclassified from stage three to stage four CKD (Salman et al. 2021). In short, the removal of the race multiplier may have implications for CKD management, treatment, and transplantation (Salman et al. 2021). In response to the debate on using a race-based algorithm, a task force was formed in 2020 by the National Kidney Foundation and the American Society of Nephrology to reassess the inclusion of race in detecting CKD (Salman et al. 2021). In 2021, the task force's final report recommended ending the inclusion of race in the eGFR calculation (Delgado et al. 2022).

1.4.2 Race-Norming and the National Football League

In 2015, the National Football League (NFL) settled a concussion class-action lawsuit with former NFL players and their families. In the suit, retired NFL football players alleged that they suffered from traumatic brain injury caused by concussion throughout their NFL careers (In Re: National Football League Players' Concussion Injury Litigation 2014). They argued that the NFL breached its duty to warn and protect the players from the long-term health effects associated with repetitive brain injuries (In Re: National Football League Players' Concussion Injury Litigation 2014). Moreover, they asserted that the NFL knew, concealed, and misrepresented the association between concussions and traumatic brain injury (In Re: National Football League Players' Concussion Injury Litigation 2014). In the settlement, the NFL agreed to create a fund of $765 million for neuropsychological and neurological exams, medical testing, counseling, treatment, monetary awards for death diagnosis with chronic traumatic encephalopathy, and educational safety and injury prevention programs for football players (In Re: National Football League Players' Concussion Injury Litigation 2014; National Football League Concussion Settlement 2023).

In 2020, two retired NFL players who were denied compensation under the settlement sued the NFL, alleging that the NFL used race correction or "race-norming" that was biased against Black players (Radnofsky and Beaton 2020). Precisely, to determine the impact of concussion, the assessment estimated the average person's performance on cognitive tests. Then, the score was adjusted for demographic factors, including race. The estimated score was lower for Blacks than Whites (Casaletto and Heaton 2017). Race was used as a proxy for social and cultural influences that may impact brain development like medical care access, education quality, and poverty, thereby affecting cognitive development (Casaletto and Heaton 2017). In application, if both a former Black player and a former White player receive identical raw scores in the cognitive functioning tests, the Black player's score will be assumed to be less cognitively impaired due to the race correction (Radnofsky and Beaton 2020).

Consequently, the race correction was scoring Black players lower, thereby precluding them from the settlement compensation. The case was dismissed in March 2020 but referred to mediation to contend with issues about the race-correction adjustment (Radnofsky and Beaton 2020). In June 2021, the NFL announced that it was ending race-norming as part of the settlement process (Hobson 2021).

1.5 Summary

Algorithms are trained on data. The lack of diversity, representation, and inclusion in data training sets may corrupt algorithmic predictions. Bias occurs when certain groups, such as racial and ethnic minority, rural, and socioeconomically disadvantaged populations, are missing from the data. The potential for bias is also perpetuated by the lack of women and racial and ethnic minorities in the technology fields because their ideas, perceptions, and values may not be represented the development, training and deployment of algorithmic tools. Moreover, race is a social construct, not a biological or genetic trait. Its inclusion may bias the algorithmic predictions. Therefore, it is crucial to investigate how race may impact algorithmic models and whether its inclusion is merited. If the data digested by the AI tools are flawed, its predictive power to identify disease and provide treatment options is equally flawed. Consequently, the promise of AI in medicine as a diagnostic tool to improve treatment outcomes, lower health care costs, and allocate resources may not be achievable unless algorithmic bias is addressed.

References

Adamson, Adewole S., and Avery Smith. 2018. Machine learning and health care disparities in dermatology. *JAMA Dermatology* 154 (11): 1247–1248.

Angwin, Julia, Jeff Larson, Surya Mattu, and Lauren Kirchner. 2016. Machine bias: There's software used across the country to predict future criminals, and it's biased against blacks. *PROPUBLICA*. https://www.propublica.org/article/machine-bias-risk-assessments-in-criminal-sentencing. Accessed July 2, 2023.

Augustus, Gaius J., and Nathan A. Ellis. 2018. Colorectal cancer disparity in African Americans: Risk factors and carcinogenic mechanisms. *The American Journal of Pathology* 188 (2): 291–303.

Bass, Dina, and Ellen Huet. 2017. Researchers combat gender and racial bias in artificial intelligence. *Bloomberg Technology*. https://www.bloomberg.com/news/articles/2017-12-04/researchers-combat-gender-and-racial-bias-in-artificial-intelligence. Accessed July 2, 2023.

Bose, Saurav, Chen C. Kenyon, and Aaron J. Masino. 2021. Personalized prediction of early childhood asthma persistence: A machine learning approach. *PLoS ONE*. https://doi.org/10.1371/journal.pone.0247784.

Branson, Richard D., Kenneth Davis, Jr., and Karyn L. Butler. 2007. African Americans' participation in clinical research: Importance, barriers, and solutions. *The American Journal of Surgery* 193 (1): 32–39.

Braun, Lundy. 2015. Race, ethnicity and lung function: A brief history. *Canadian Journal of Respiratory Therapy Fall* 51 (4): 99–101.

Broussard, Meredith. 2018. *Artificial unintelligence: How computers misunderstand the world*. Cambridge: The MIT Press.

Buolamwini, J., and T. Gebru. 2018. Gender shades: Intersectional accuracy disparities in commercial gender classification. *Proceedings of Machine Learning Research* 81: 77–91.

Bustamante, Carlos, Francisco M. De La Vega, and Esteban G. Burchard. 2011. Genomics for the world. *Nature* 475: 163–165.

Campolo, Alex, Madelyn Sanfilippo, Meredith Whittaker, and Kate Crawford. 2017. AI Now 2017 report. *AI NOW*, 13–21. https://ainowinstitute.org/publication/ai-now-2017-report-2. Accessed

July 2, 2023.
Casaletto, Kaitlin B., and Robert K. Heaton. 2017. Neuropsychological assessment: Past and future. *Journal of the International Neuropsychological Society* 23 (9–10): 778–790.
Cerdeña Jessica, P., Marie V. Plaisime, and Jennifer Tsai. 2020. From race-based to race-conscious medicine: How anti-racist uprisings call us to act. *Lancet* 396 (10257): 1125–1128.
Dastin, Jeffrey. 2018. Amazon scraps secret AI recruiting tool that showed bias against women. *Reuters*. https://www.reuters.com/article/us-amazon-com-jobs-automation-insight/amazon-scraps-secret-ai-recruiting-tool-that-showed-bias-against-women-idUSKCN1MK08G. Accessed July 2, 2023.
Datta, Amit, Michael Carl Tschantz, and Anupam Datta. 2015. Automated experiments on ad privacy settings: A tale of opacity, choice and discrimination. *Proceedings on Privacy Enhancing Technologies* 1: 92–112.
Delgado, Cynthia, Mukta Baweja, Nilka Ríos Burrows, Deidra C. Crews, Nwamaka D. Eneanya, Crystal A. Gadegbeku, Lesley A. Inker, Mallika L. Mendu, W. Greg Miller, Marva M. Moxey-Mims, Glenda V. Roberts, Wendy L. St. Peter, Curtis Warfield, and Neil R. Powe. 2021. Reassessing the inclusion of race in diagnosing kidney diseases: An interim report from the NKF-ASN task force. *Journal of the American Society of Nephrology* 32 (6): 1305–1317.
Delgado, Cynthia, Mukta Baweja, Deidra C. Crews, Nwamaka D. Eneanya, Crystal A. Gadegbeku, Lesley A. Inker, Mallika L. Mendu, W. Greg Miller, Marva M. Moxey-Mims, Glenda V. Roberts, Wendy L. St. Peter, Curtis Warfield, and Neil R. Powe. 2022. A Unifying approach for GFR estimation: Recommendations of the NKF-ASN task force on reassessing the inclusion of race in diagnosing kidney disease. *American Journal of Kidney Disease* 79 (2): 268–288.
Domingos, Pedro. 2015. *The master algorithm: How the quest for the ultimate machine will make our world*. New York, NY: Basic Books.
Dressel, Julia, and Hany Farid. 2018. The accuracy, fairness, and limits of predicting recidivism. *Science Advances* 4 (1): 1–5.
Eshaghi, Arman, Alexandria L. Young, Peter A. Wijeratne, Ferran Prados, Douglas L. Arnold, Sridar Narayanan, Charles R.G. Guttmann, Frederik Barkhof, Daniel C. Alexander, Alan J. Thompson, Declan Chard, and Olga Ciccarelli. 2021. Identifying multiple sclerosis subtypes using unsupervised machine learning and MRI data. *Nature Communications* 12 (1): 2078.
Executive Office of the President. 2014. Big data: Seizing opportunities, preserving values. https://obamawhitehouse.archives.gov/sites/default/files/docs/big_data_privacy_report_5.1.14_final_print.pdf. Accessed August 9, 2023.
Gandomi, Amir, and Murtaza Haider. 2015. Beyond the hype: Big data concepts, methods, and analytics. *International Journal of Information Management* 35: 137–144.
Garvie, Claire, and Jonathan Frankle. 2016. Facial-recognition software might have a racial bias problem. *The Atlantic*. https://www.theatlantic.com/technology/archive/2016/04/the-underlying-bias-of-facial-recognition-systems/476991/. Accessed August 14, 2023.
Grobman, Williams A., Grecio Sandoval, Madeline Murguia Rice, Monica Longo, and Mark B. Landon. 2021. Prediction of vaginal birth after cesarean delivery in term gestations: A calculator without race and ethnicity. *American Journal of Obstetrics and Gynecology*. https://doi.org/10.1016/j.ajog.2021.05.021.
Guynn, Jessica. 2015. Google photos labeled black people 'gorillas.' *USA Today*. https://www.usatoday.com/story/tech/2015/07/01/google-apologizes-after-photos-identify-black-people-as-gorillas/29567465/. Accessed July 2, 2023.
Hansen, M.M., T. Miron-Shatz, A.Y.S. Lau, and C. Paton. 2014. Big data in science and healthcare: A review of recent literature and perspectives. Contribution of the IMIA social media working group. *Yearbook of Medical Informatics* 9 (1): 21–26.
Himes, Deborah O., Aubri E. Root, Amanda Gammon, and Karlen E. Luthy. 2016. Breast cancer risk assessment: Calculating lifetime risk using the Tyrer–Cuzick model. *The Journal for Nurse Practitioners* 12(9): 581–592.

Hobson, Will. 2021. NFL says it will end controversial "race-norming" in concussion settlement with players. *The Washington Post*. https://www.washingtonpost.com/sports/2021/06/03/nfl-concussion-settlement-race-norming/. Accessed August 9, 2023.

Ingold, David, and Spencer Soper. 2016. Amazon doesn't consider the race of its customers. Should it? *Bloomberg*. https://www.bloomberg.com/graphics/2016-amazon-same-day/. Accessed July 2, 2023.

In Re: National Football League Players' Concussion Injury Litigation. 2014. MDL No. 2323. https://www.nflconcussionsettlement.com/Docs/Amended%20Class%20Action.pdf. Accessed August 9, 2023.

IT Modernization Centers of Excellence. n.d. AI guide for government. A living and evolving guide to the application of artificial intelligence for the U.S. federal government. https://coe.gsa.gov/coe/ai-guide-for-government/what-is-ai-key-terminology/. Accessed August 9, 2023.

Kaba, R., and P. Sooriakumaran. 2007. The evolution of the doctor-patient relationship. *International Journal of Surgery* 5 (1): 57–65.

Karr, Alan, Ashish P. Sanil, and David L. Banks. 2002. *Data quality: A statistical perspective*. National Institute of Statistical Sciences. https://www.niss.org/sites/default/files/technicalreports/tr129.pdf. Accessed September 11, 2023.

Knight, Will. 2017. Biased algorithms are everywhere, and no one seems to care. *MIT Technology Review*. https://www.technologyreview.com/s/608248/biased-algorithms-are-everywhere-and-no-one-seems-to-care/. Accessed July 2, 2023.

Krittanawong, Chayakrit, HongJu Zhang, Zhen Wang, Mehmet Aydar, and Takeshi Kitai. 2017. Artificial intelligence in precision cardiovascular medicine. *Journal of the American College of Cardiology* 69 (21): 2657–2664.

Larson, Jeff, Surya Mattau, Lauren Kirchner, and Julia Angwin. 2016. How we analyzed the COMPAS recidivism algorithm. *ProPublica*. https://www.propublica.org/article/how-we-analyzed-the-compas-recidivism-algorithm. Accessed July 2, 2023.

Livingston, Steven, and Mathias Risse. 2019. The future impact of artificial intelligence on humans and human rights. *Ethics & International Affairs* 33 (2): 141–158.

Lujan, Heidi L., and Stephen E. DiCarlo. 2018. Science reflects history as society influences science: Brief history of "race", "race correction", and the spirometer. *Advances in Physiology Education* 42: 163–165.

Maddalena, Favaretto, Eva De Clercq, Christophe Schneble, and Bernice Simone Elger. 2020. What is your definition of big data? Researchers' understanding of the phenomenon of the decade. *PLoS ONE* 15 (2): e0228987.

Matheny, Michael, Soon Thadaney Israni, Mahnoor Ahmed, and Danielle Whicher. 2019. *Artificial intelligence in health care: The hope, the hype, the promise, the peril*. NAM Special Publication. Washington, DC: National Academy of Medicine.

Mayo Clinic. 2021. *C-section*. https://www.mayoclinic.org/tests-procedures/c-section/about/pac-20393655. Accessed July 2, 2023.

McCorduck, Pamela. 2018. *Machines who think*. New York: CRC Press.

Mehrabi, Ninreh, Fred Morstatter, Nripusuta Saxena, Kristina Lerman, and Aram Galstyan. 2021. A survey on bias and fairness in machine learning. *ACM Computing Surveys* 54 (6): 115, 1–35.

Moor, James. 2006. The Dartmouth college artificial intelligence conference: The next fifty years. *AI Magazine* 27 (4): 87–91.

National Football League Concussion Settlement. 2023. In Re: National Football League players' concussion injury litigation, MDL No. 2323. Basic Information. https://www.nflconcussionsettlement.com/FAQDetails.aspx?q=155#15. Accessed August 9, 2023.

National Science Foundation. 2022. The state of U.S. science and engineering 2022. https://ncses.nsf.gov/pubs/nsb20221/u-s-and-global-stem-education-and-labor-force. Accessed July 2, 2023.

National Science and Technology Council, Committee on Technology. 2016. *Preparing for the future of artificial intelligence*. Executive Office of the President. https://obamawhitehouse.archives.gov/sites/default/files/whitehouse_files/microsites/ostp/NSTC/preparing_for_the_future_of_ai.pdf. Accessed July 2, 2023.

Naudé, Wim, and Nicola Dimitri. 2019. The race for an artificial general intelligence: Implications for public policy. *AI & Society* 35 (2): 367–379.

Need, Anna C., and David B. Goldstein. 2009. Next generation disparities in human genomics: Concerns and remedies. *Trends in Genetics* 25 (11): 489–494.

Nilsson, Nils J. 2010. *Quest for artificial intelligence.* New York: Cambridge University Press.

Obermeyer, Ziad, Brian Powers, Christine Vogeli, and Sendhil Mullainathan. 2019. Dissecting racial bias in an algorithm used to manage the health of populations. *Science* 366 (6464): 447–453.

O'Neil, Cathy. 2016. *Weapons of math destruction.* New York: Broadway Books.

O'Reilly-Shah, Vikas N., Katherine R. Gentry, Andrew M. Walters, Joal Zivot, Corrie T. Anderson, and Patrick J. Tighe. 2020. Bias and ethical considerations in machine learning and the automation of perioperative risk assessment. *British Journal of Anaesthesia* 125 (6): 843–846.

Palmer, Katie. 2021. Changing the equation: Researchers remove race from a calculator for childbirth. *STAT.* https://www.statnews.com/2021/06/03/vbac-calculator-birth-cesarean/?utm_source=STAT+Newsletters&utm_campaign=6009a9773a-Daily_Recap&utm_medium=e. Accessed August 9, 2023.

Peek, N., J.H. Holmes, and J. Sun. 2014. Technical challenges for big data in biomedicine and health: Data sources, infrastructure, and analytics. *Yearbook of Medical Informatics* 9 (1): 42–47.

Popejoy, Alice B., and Stephanie M. Fullerton. 2016. Genomics is failing diversity. *Nature* 538 (7624): 161–164.

Radnofsky, Louise, and Andrew Beaton. 2020. Lawsuit allege NFL's concussion settlement discriminates against black players. *The Wall Street Journal.* https://www.wsj.com/articles/lawsuit-alleges-nfls-concussion-settlement-discriminates-against-black-players-11598371843. Accessed September 10, 2023.

Robbins, Rebecca, and Erin Brodwin. 2020. An invisible hand: Patients aren't being told about the AI systems advising their care. *STAT.* https://www.statnews.com/2020/07/15/artificial-intelligence-patient-consent-hospitals/. Accessed August 9, 2023.

Russell, Stuart J., and Peter Norvig. 2010. *Artificial intelligence: Modern approach*, 3rd ed. New Jersey: Prentice-Hall.

Salman, Ahmed, Cameron T. Nutt, Nwamaka D. Eneanya, Peter P. Reese, Karthik Sivashanker, Michelle Morse, Thomas Sequis, and Mallika L. Mendu. 2021. Examining the potential impact of race multiplier utilization in estimated glomerular filtration rate calculation on African American care outcomes. *Journal of General Internal Medicine* 36 (2): 464–471.

Scherer, Matthew U. 2016. Regulating artificial intelligence systems: Risks, challenges, competencies, and strategies. *Harvard Journal of Law & Technology* 29: 360–361.

Smith, Jacque, and Cassie Spodak. 2021. Black or other? Doctors may be relying on race to make decisions about your health. *CNN.* https://www.cnn.com/2021/04/25/health/race-correction-in-medicine-history-refocused/index.html. Accessed August 9, 2023.

The National Coordination Office for Networking and Information Technology Research and Development (NITRD/NCO). 2016. The federal big data research and development strategic plan. https://www.nitrd.gov/PUBS/bigdatardstrategicplan.pdf. Accessed July 2, 2023.

The Society for Women's Health Research and the U.S. Food and Drug Administration Office of Women's Health. 2011. Dialogues on diversifying clinical trials: Successful strategies for engaging women and minorities in clinical trials. https://www.fda.gov/files/science%20&%20research/published/White-Paper-on-the-Dialogues-on-Diversifying-Clinical-Trials-Conference.pdf. Accessed July 2, 2023.

The White House. Office of Science and Technology Policy. 2022. Blueprint for an AI bill of rights. https://www.whitehouse.gov/ostp/ai-bill-of-rights/. Accessed July 24, 2023.

U.S. Census Bureau. 2023. QuickFacts population estimates, July 1, 2022. https://www.census.gov/quickfacts/fact/table/US/PST045222. Accessed August 16, 2023.

U.S. Department of Health and Human Services. 2023. Artificial intelligence (AI) at HHS. https://www.hhs.gov/about/agencies/asa/ocio/ai/index.html. Accessed August 9, 2023.

U.S. Department of Health and Human Services. Agency for Healthcare Research and Quality. 2021. Use of clinical algorithms that have the potential to introduce racial/ethnic bias into healthcare delivery. https://effectivehealthcare.ahrq.gov/products/algorithms-bias-healthcare-delivery. Accessed August 9, 2023.

U.S. Department of Health and Human Services. Agency for Healthcare Research and Quality. 2023. Research protocol: Impact of healthcare algorithms on racial and ethnic disparities in health and healthcare. https://effectivehealthcare.ahrq.gov/products/racial-disparities-health-healthcare/protocol. Accessed July 3, 2023.

U.S. Department of Health and Human Services, Centers for Disease Control and Prevention. 2023. Chronic kidney disease in the United States, 2023. https://www.cdc.gov/kidneydisease/pdf/CKD-Factsheet-H.pdf. Accessed August 9, 2023.

U.S. Department of Health and Human Services. National Human Genome Research Institute. 2021. Genome-wide association studies (GWAS). https://www.genome.gov/genetics-glossary/Genome-Wide-Association-Studies#:~:text=A%20genome%2Dwide%20association%20study,the%20presence%20of%20a%20disease. Accessed August 9, 2023.

U.S. Department of Health and Human Services. National Institutes of Health. 2017. NIH policy and guidelines on the inclusion of women and minorities as subjects in clinical research. https://grants.nih.gov/grants/funding/women_min/guidelines.htm. Accessed July 2, 2023.

U.S. Food and Drug Administration. 2018. FDA permits marketing of artificial intelligence-based device to detect certain diabetes-related eye problems. https://www.fda.gov/news-events/press-announcements/fda-permits-marketing-artificial-intelligence-based-device-detect-certain-diabetes-related-eye. Accessed July 2, 2023.

U.S. Food and Drug Administration. 2021. Authorizes marketing of first device that uses artificial intelligence to help detect potential signs of colon cancer. https://www.fda.gov/news-events/press-announcements/fda-authorizes-marketing-first-device-uses-artificial-intelligence-help-detect-potential-signs-colon. Accessed July 2, 2023.

U.S. Government Accountability Office. 2023. Science and tech spotlight: Generative AI. https://www.gao.gov/products/gao-23-106782#:~:text=Generative%20artificial%20intelligence%20(AI)%20is,and%20images%20from%20the%20internet. Accessed August 9, 2023.

Van Poucke, Sven, Michiel Thomeer, and Admir Hadzic. 2015. Big data in healthcare: For whom the bell tolls? *Critical Care* 19 (1): 171.

Vickers, Selwyn M., and Mona N. Fouad. 2014. An overview of EMPaCT and fundamental issues affecting minority participation in cancer clinical trials: Enhancing minority participation in clinical trials (EMPaCT): Laying the groundwork for improving minority clinical trial accrual. *Cancer* 120 (Suppl 7): 1087–1090.

Vyas, Darshali, David S. Jones, Audra R. Meadows, Khady Diouf, Nawal M. Nour, and Julianna Schantz-Dunn. 2019. Challenging the use of race in the vaginal birth after cesarean section calculator. *Women's Health Issues* 29 (3): 201–204.

Vyas, Darshali A., Leo G. Eisenstein, and David S. Jones. 2020. Hidden in plain sight—Reconsidering the use of race correction in clinical algorithms. *New England Journal of Medicine* 383 (9): 874–882.

Washington, Harriet A. 2006. *Medical apartheid: The dark history of medical experimentation on Black Americans from colonial times to the present*. New York: Anchor Books.

Williams, Natasha H. 2019. *Exploring the potential of artificial intelligence to improve minority health and reduce health disparities*. National Institute on Minority Health and Health Disparities. https://blog.nimhd.nih.gov/archives-2019/news_feed/exploring-the-potential-of-artificial-intelligence-to-improve-minority-health-and-reduce-health-disparities. Accessed August 9, 2023.

Williams, Betsy Ann, Catherine F. Brooks, and Yotam Shmargad. 2018. How algorithms discriminate based on data they lack: Challenges, solutions, and policy implications. *Journal of Information Policy* 8: 78–115.

Zhang, Xinzhi, Eliseo J. Pérez-Stable, Philip E. Bourne, Emmanual Peprah, O. Kenrik Duru, Nancy Breen, David Berrigan, Fred Wood, James S. Jackson, David W.S. Wong, and Joshua Denny. 2017. Big data science: Opportunities and challenges to address minority health and health disparities in the 21st century. *Ethnicity & Disease* 27 (2): 95–106.

Chapter 2
What Are Health Disparities?

Abstract Many racial and ethnic minority groups have poor health outcomes. These health disparities are driven by the social determinants of health. The social determinants of health are where people live, work, and play. Algorithms also impact where we live, work, and play. Section 2.1 describes health disparities and their economic costs. Section 2.2 explains the social determinants of health and their impact on health. Section 2.3 justifies algorithmic bias as a social determinant of health. Section 2.4 summarizes key points in the chapter.

Keywords Health disparities · Health equity · Social determinants of health · Algorithms · Obesity · Hypertension

2.1 Definition of Health Disparities

Released in 1985, the *Report of the Secretary's Task Force on Black and Minority Health* was the result of the first U.S. government-led task force of health experts to study racial and ethnic minority health (Gracia 2018; U.S. Department of Health and Human Services. Margaret M. Heckler 1985). This landmark report was also known as the Heckler Report, after the former U.S. Department of Health and Human Services Secretary Margaret H. Heckler, who led the effort. Secretary Heckler wrote,

> … there was a continuing disparity in the burden of death and illness experienced by Blacks and other minority Americans as compared with our nation's population as a whole. That disparity has existed ever since accurate federal record keeping began—more than a generation ago. And although our health charts do itemize steady gains in the health status of minority Americans, the stubborn disparity remained—an affront both to our ideals and to the ongoing genius of American medicine. I felt passionately—that it was time to decipher the message inherent in that disparity. In order to unravel the complex picture provided by our data and experience, I established a Secretarial Task Force whose broad assignment was the comprehensive investigation of the health problems of Blacks, Native Americans, Hispanics and Asian/Pacific Islanders. (U.S. Department of Health and Human Services. Margaret M. Heckler 1985, p. ix)

N. H. Williams, *Artificial Intelligence and Healthcare*, The International Library of Bioethics 107, https://doi.org/10.1007/978-3-031-48262-5_2

The Heckler Report was a comprehensive analysis and synthesis of the significant health facts that impacted the health status of these communities of color (U.S. Department of Health and Human Services. Margaret M. Heckler 1985). It raised health disparities and minority health into the national consciousness. Based upon analysis of mortality data from 1979 to 1981, the report identified "six causes of death that together account for more than 80% of the mortality observed among Blacks and other minority groups in excess of that in the White population" (U.S. Department of Health and Human Services. Margaret M. Heckler 1985, p. 3). These were "cancer, cardiovascular disease and stroke, chemical dependence (measured by deaths due to cirrhosis), diabetes, homicide and accidents, and infant mortality" (U.S. Department of Health and Human Services. Margaret M. Heckler 1985, p. 4). For each identified cause of death, the task force studied the cause of each condition, identified intervention strategies, and explored improvements to treatment (U.S. Department of Health and Human Services. Margaret M. Heckler 1985). Recommendations included launching a health education outreach campaign; ensuring patient education is responsive to the needs of minority populations; training health professionals to be perceptive of cultural and linguistic needs; developing and implementing models of health services delivery and financing; creating strategies to improve the accessibility of health professionals in minority communities; building capacity in State, local, and community organizations to address minority health needs; improving sources of health data; and developing a research agenda that examines factors that impact minority health (U.S. Department of Health and Human Services. Margaret M. Heckler 1985).

In another milestone study by the Institute of Medicine titled *Unequal Treatment: Confronting Racial and Ethnic Disparities in Health Care*,[1] the authors defined disparities in health care "as racial or ethnic differences in the quality of healthcare that are not due to access-related factors or clinical needs, preferences, and appropriateness of intervention" (Institute of Medicine (U.S.) Committee on Understanding and Eliminating Racial and Ethnic Disparities in Health Care 2003, p. 32). The National Institutes of Health (NIH) describes a health disparity as "a health difference that adversely affects disadvantaged populations, based on one or more of the following health outcomes: (1) higher incidence and/or prevalence and earlier onset of disease; (2) higher prevalence of risk factors, unhealthy behaviors, or clinical measures in the causal pathway of a disease outcome; (3) higher rates of condition-specific symptoms, reduced global daily functioning, or self-reported health-related quality of life using standardized measures; (4) premature and/or excessive mortality from diseases where population rates differ; and (5) greater global burden of disease using a standardized metric" (U.S. Department of Health and Human Services.

[1] The National Academy of Medicine (NAM) was founded as the Institute of Medicine (IOM) in 1970. IOM's name was changed in 2015 to NAM. NAM, the National Academy of Sciences, and the National Academy of Engineering comprise the National Academies in the United States. The National Academics are nonprofit, private organizations that provide independent and expert scientific advice to inform policy.

National Institutes of Health 2021, p. 6). In Healthy People 2030,[2] a health disparity is defined as a "particular type of health difference that was closely linked with social, economic, and/or environmental disadvantage. Health disparities adversely affected groups of people who have systematically experienced greater obstacles to health based on their racial or ethnic group; religion; socioeconomic status; gender; age; mental health; cognitive, sensory, or physical disability; sexual orientation or gender identity; geographic location; or other characteristics historically linked to discrimination or exclusion" (U.S. Department of Health and Human Services. Office of the Assistant Secretary for Health. Office of Disease Prevention and Health Promotion 2022, p. 31). Despite the definitional differences, the common theme is that health disparities are differences between groups in the burden of disease, death, and quality of care.

Health disparities and health inequities are often used interchangeably, but they are different concepts. The World Health Organization refers to health inequities as "systematic differences in the health status of different population groups. These inequities have significant social and economic costs both to individuals and societies. Health inequities are differences in health status or in the distribution of health resources between different population groups, arising from the social conditions in which people are born, grow, live, work and age. Health inequities are unfair and could be reduced by the right mix of government policies" (World Health Organization 2018). When comparing the two, health disparities are health differences that adversely impact a group, whereas health inequity occurs when there is not equal access, utilization, and quality of care for all (Whitehead 1992).

Health disparities are complex and multifaceted. They involve biological, behavioral, environmental, socioeconomic, and cultural factors across the life course. Health disparities are influenced not only by individual aspects, but also community, societal, and political factors (U.S. Department of Health and Human Services. National Institutes of Health 2021). In the United States, populations that experience health disparities are racial and ethnic minorities[3]; socioeconomically disadvantaged populations; underserved rural populations; sexual and gender minorities; and people with disabilities (U.S. Department of Health and Human Services. National Institutes of Health 2021).[4] Many of these populations fall behind Whites in life expectancy

---

[2] Healthy People 2030 is a United States health initiative that identified health priorities to improve health and well-being. Every decade, Healthy People makes changes to the initiative based upon feedback from individuals and organizations. https://health.gov/healthypeople/about#:~:text=Whatpercent20ispercent20Healthypercent20Peoplepercent202030,overpercent20thepercent20firstpercent204percent20decades.

[3] In this book, racial and ethnic group classifications are adopted from the U.S. Office of Management and Budget Statistical Policy Directive No. 15: *Standards for Maintaining, Collecting, and Presenting Federal Data on Race and Ethnicity*. These the classification are: African American or Black; American Indian and Alaska Native; Asian; Native Hawaiian and Other Pacific Islander, and White. Ethnicity is Hispanic or Latino.

[4] For research supported by the National Institutes of Health (NIH), populations that experience health disparities are designated by the director of the National Institute on Minority Health and Health Disparities at NIH in consultation with the director of the Agency for Healthcare Research and Quality. Such a designation promotes research focused on the health and health outcomes of the

and chronic health conditions. Life expectancy "represents the average number of years a group of infants would live if they were to experience throughout life the age-specific death rates prevailing during a period" (Arias et al. 2022, p. 1). In 2021, the life expectancy in the United States was 76.1 years, a decline from 77.0 years in 2020 (Arias et al. 2022). For Whites, life expectancy was 76.4 years, Blacks 70.8 years, and American Indians and Alaska Natives, 65.2 years (Arias et al. 2022). On the other hand, the life expectancy for the Hispanic (77.7 years) and Asian (83.5 years) populations was higher than the White population (Arias et al. 2022). An analysis of trends in mortality rates for the leading causes of death from 1999 to 2015 found:

> In 2015, blacks had 40% higher death rates than whites for all-cause mortality in all age groups <65 years (Table 4). At ages 18–34 years, blacks had higher death rates than whites for eight of the 10 leading causes of death among blacks in that age group (heart disease; cancer; cerebrovascular disease; diabetes mellitus; homicide; HIV disease; and conditions resulting from pregnancy, childbirth, and the puerperium). At ages 35–49 years, blacks had higher death rates than whites for heart disease; cancer; cerebrovascular disease; diabetes mellitus; homicide; nephritis, nephrotic syndrome, and nephrosis; septicemia; and HIV disease. At ages 50–64 years, blacks had higher death rates than whites for leading chronic diseases (heart disease, cancer; cerebrovascular disease; diabetes mellitus; and nephritis, nephrotic syndrome, and nephrosis) as well as for unintentional injury, septicemia, and HIV disease. (Cunningham et al. 2017, p. 446)

Moreover, the analysis found that Blacks, when compared to Whites, were more likely to report fair to poor health status, the inability to see a doctor due to the cost during the last year, and taking medication to control high blood pressure (Cunningham et al. 2017).

Health inequalities have a social and economic cost to society due to expenditures associated with illness, premature death, family leave, and work productivity. Drs. Thomas LaVeist, Darrel Gaskin, and Patrick Richard estimated the economic cost of health inequalities in the United States (LaVeist et al. 2011). They determined that between 2003 and 2006, 30.6% of direct medical costs incurred by Blacks, Hispanics, and Asians were due to health inequalities (LaVeist et al. 2011). Moreover, eliminating health inequalities would reduce direct medical care costs by approximately $229 billion (LaVeist et al. 2011). Of those excess costs, Blacks represented more than 59% ($135.9 billion), Hispanics 35.7% ($82.0 billion), and Asians 5% ($11.4 billion) (LaVeist et al. 2011).

In addition, the researchers calculated the indirect costs associated with eliminating health inequalities. Indirect costs included the loss of individual productivity and premature death (LaVeist et al. 2011). For example, someone who was ill would not be able to work to their full potential or work at all. The illness may have incurred associated medical costs like insurance co-pays, nursing support, medication, medical transport, and home health assistance, which further impact the household finances. Those monies once allocated toward household costs were reallocated to medical bills. If a wage earner or someone who contributes to the household (e.g., a retiree) died, the household experienced financial adjustments because that

designated populations. In September 2023, people with disabilities were designated as a population with health disparities.

individual's income no longer existed (LaVeist et al. 2011). It may have resulted in housing and financial insecurity and role adjustment in the household, not to mention the emotional distress and anxiety associated with the personal loss (LaVeist et al. 2011). There are many stories of families whose loved one died or became ill, and they could no longer afford to live in their home or community (LaVeist et al. 2011). The indirect costs due of health inequities due to premature death were $957.5 billion and $50.3 billion from illness (LaVeist et al. 2011). Of the indirect costs due to health inequities, which included both premature death and illness, Blacks represented 77%, Hispanics 22.3% and Asians 0.03% (LaVeist et al. 2011).

In a 2023 analysis, the problem had not improved (LaVeist et al. 2023). The study estimated the total economic burden of health disparities nationally, at the state level, and for the following racial and ethnic minorities: Asians, American Indians/Alaska Natives, Blacks/African Americans, Hispanics/Latinos, and Native Hawaiians/Pacific Islanders (LaVeist et al. 2023). The researchers also estimated the total economic burden of health disparities for "adults with less than high school/general educational development test (GED), adults with high school/GED, and adults with some college" (U.S. Department of Health and Human Services. National Institutes of Health. National Institute on Minority Health and Health Disparities 2023). They examined excess medical care costs, lost labor market productivity, and premature deaths. The researchers found that in 2018, "racial and ethnic health disparities cost the U.S. economy $451 billion, a 41% increase from the previous estimate of $320 billion in 2014. The study also finds that the total burden of education-related health disparities for persons with less than a college degree in 2018 reached $978 billion, about two times greater than the annual growth rate of the U.S. economy in 2018" (U.S. Department of Health and Human Services. National Institutes of Health 2023). Nationally, researchers found:

> Most of the economic burden for racial and ethnic disparities was borne by Black/African American population (69%) due to the level of premature mortality. Native Hawaiian/Pacific Islander ($23,225) and American Indian/Alaska Native ($12,351) populations had the highest economic burden per person. Most of the economic burden was attributed to premature deaths for Native Hawaiian/Pacific Islander (90%), Black/African American (77%), and American Indian/Alaska Native (74%) populations. For Asian (55%) and Hispanic/Latino (43%) populations, most of the burden was from excess medical care costs and lost labor market productivity, respectively … Per person, adults with a high school diploma had the highest burden ($9,982), followed closely by adults with less than a high school diploma ($9,467) and then adults with some college ($2,028). Although most of the burden of education-related health inequities was borne by adults with a high school diploma/GED (61%), a disproportionate share was borne by adults with less than a high school diploma/GED—they were only 9% of the population but bore 26% of the burden. Across all educational levels, most of the burden was attributable to premature deaths (66%), followed by lost labor market productivity (18%) and excess medical care costs (16%). (U.S. Department of Health and Human Services. National Institutes of Health 2023)

To remedy these disparities, the researchers recommended that policymakers develop policies and programs that address inequity, structural barriers, and socioeconomic inequalities (LaVeist et al. 2023).

2.2 The Social Determinants of Health

The World Health Organization defines the social determinants of health (SDOH) as "the conditions in which people are born, grow, work, live, and age, and the wider set of forces and systems shaping the conditions of daily life. These forces and systems include economic policies and systems, development agendas, social norms, social policies, and political systems. Social determinants of health are mostly responsible for health inequities—the unfair and avoidable differences in health status seen within and between countries" (World Health Organization 2021). Similarly, the Centers for Disease Control and Prevention describes SDOH as the circumstances where people work, live, play, and learn (U.S. Department of Health and Human Services. Centers for Disease Control and Prevention 2021). They include "health care access and quality, education access and quality, social and community context, economic stability, and neighborhood and built environment" (U.S. Department of Health and Human Services. Centers for Disease Control and Prevention 2021).

Social, environmental, and socioeconomic factors impact health and health outcomes such as access to health insurance, quality health care, employment, housing, and income. The SDOH falls into five categories. These are health care access and quality, education access and quality, social and community context, socioeconomic factors, and neighborhood and built environment (see Fig. 2.1). These

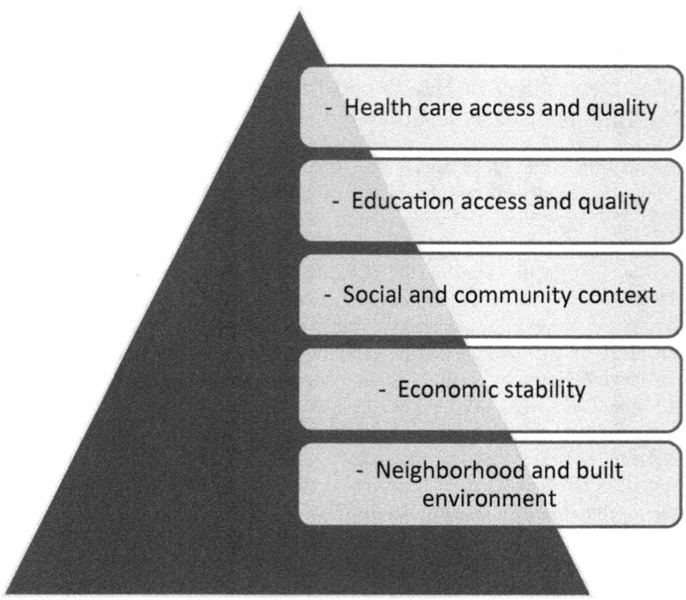

Fig. 2.1 The social determinants of health

determinants have a societal impact, especially for racial and ethnic minority populations (U.S. Department of Health and Human Services. Centers for Disease Control and Prevention 2021).

2.2.1 Health Care Access and Quality

Health care access and quality equates to people being able to obtain the health services they need. In 2021, 27.2 million people in the United States did not have health insurance (Keisler-Starkey and Bunch 2022). Health insurance impacts not only the ability to pay for medical care, but also access to quality care (Keisler-Starkey and Bunch 2022). The lack of health insurance affects the type of health care and providers that people can access. Additionally, people who are underinsured—having insufficient medical coverage—may have higher out-of-pocket medical costs (Keisler-Starkey and Bunch 2022). In a study examining the impact of health insurance coverage on children with asthma, the researchers found that health coverage was associated with cost barriers to care (Pate et al. 2020). Specifically, uninsured and partially insured children faced cost barriers in seeing a doctor and buying medication than those with full insurance; Black children with insurance experienced cost barriers to visiting a doctor compared to White children; and those children with public insurance experienced a cost barrier to seeing a doctor when compared to those on private insurance (Pate et al. 2020).

Many people live in medical deserts, which are areas where certain medical services are limited or completely absent. For example, nearly half of rural community hospitals in the United States did not provide obstetric services in 2020, and approximately over two million women of childbearing age lived in maternity care deserts (March of Dimes 2022). These are areas that have limited or no access to maternity care. In 2020, in the United States, there were over 19,000 infant deaths (Ely and Driscoll 2020).[5] In a 2018 analysis examining the leading causes of infant death in the United States from 2013 to 2015, researchers found that infant mortality was higher in rural counties than in small, medium, and large urban counties (Ely and Hoyert 2018). Moreover, neonatal mortality (i.e., death during the first 28 days) rates were higher in rural counties than in large urban counties (Ely and Hoyert 2018). Post-neonatal mortality (i.e., death between 29 and 364 days of life) was higher in rural counties than in small, medium, and large urban counties (Ely and Hoyert 2018; Ely and Driscoll 2020).

[5] In 2020, the U.S. infant mortality rate was 5.42 deaths per 1000 live births. In 2020, the infant mortality rate was highest among Black women (10.38), American Indian/Alaska Native (7.68), Native Hawaiian or Other Pacific Islander (7.17), Hispanic (4.69), White (4.40), and Asian (3.14).

2.2.2 Education Access and Quality

People with higher educational attainment have better health outcomes than those who are less educated (LaVeist et al. 2023; Zajacova and Lawrence 2018). Early childhood poverty can impact educational outcomes for children, decreasing a child's readiness for school (Karoly et al. 2005). Compared to their wealthier counterparts, these children experience stressors such substandard housing, pollution, violence, familial conflict, and limited access to green spaces and healthy food choices (Evans and Kim 2013). Additionally, impoverished neighborhoods have limited resources, which impact classroom quality and academic achievement (Lacour and Tissington 2011).

2.2.3 Social and Community Context

Social engagement and interpersonal relationships with family, co-workers, and friends within their community (U.S. Department of Health and Human Services. Centers for Disease Control and Prevention 2021) is a SDOH. It is the sense of belonging, well-being, security, and social cohesion within the community. It involves people having social support, feeling safe where they live and work, and developing positive relationships. Discrimination and racism impact that feeling of belonging, safety, social support, and positive relationships (U.S. Department of Health and Human Services. Centers for Disease Control and Prevention 2021). Hypertension is a silent killer and can lead to stroke, vision loss, heart failure, heart attack, and kidney disease and failure (American Heart Association 2016).[6] From 2017 to 2018, the prevalence of hypertension in the United States was 45.4%. Blacks had the highest prevalence of hypertension (57.1%) followed by Hispanics (43.7.%) and Whites (43.6%) (Ostchega et al. 2021). Researchers studied whether everyday discrimination, lifetime discrimination, and stress were associated with hypertension (Forde et al. 2020). The study found that lifetime discrimination may increase the risk of hypertension because it is a chronic stressor (Forde et al. 2020).

2.2.4 Economic Stability

Poverty, educational attainment, and household income impact economic stability. In 2021, 37.9 million people were living in poverty (Creamer et al. 2022). The poverty rate for non-Hispanic Whites was 8.1%, 24.3% for American Indians and Alaska Natives, 19.5% for Blacks, 17.1% for Hispanics, and 9.3% for Asians (Creamer et al.

[6] Stage 1 hypertension is a systolic pressure of 130–139 or a diastolic pressure of 80–89. Stage 2 hypertension is a systolic pressure of 140 or higher or diastolic pressure of 90 or higher (American Heart Association 2016).

2022). In 2021, more females (12.6%) lived in poverty than males (10.5%). Moreover, "the poverty rate for those without a high school diploma was 27.2%, six-and-a-half times higher than those with at least a bachelor's degree (4.1%). People with a bachelor's degree or higher had the lowest poverty rate of the educational attainment groups" (Creamer et al. 2022, p. 6). In 2021, the real[7] U.S. median household income was $70,784 (Semega and Kollar 2022). The median income for Black households was $48,297, $77,999 for White, not Hispanic, households, $57,981 for Hispanic households, and $101,418 for Asian households (Semega and Kollar 2022).

2.2.5 *Neighborhood and Built Environment*

The neighborhood and built environment refer to the structures and community amenities such as walking trails, recreational facilities, grocery stores, and healthy food choices that may affect health behavior. They also include environmental impacts (U.S. Department of Health and Human Services. Centers for Disease Control and Prevention 2021). For instance, does someone live in a home with lead paint, or in a neighborhood near a factory or busy highway? Does the neighborhood have healthy food choices, or is it in a food desert? Do residents feel safe to go for a walk? Is there access to internet service? These are a few examples of how the neighborhood and built environment impact health. Researchers examined hypertension disparities between Black and White adults that lived in gentrifying communities (Smith et al. 2020).[8] In their final analysis, researchers found that the prevalence of hypertension among Blacks living in gentrified communities was no different than that of Whites living in gentrified communities. In short, the prevalence of hypertension was similar between the races (Smith et al. 2020). Researchers attributed this to the impact of the environment in which people lived (Smith et al. 2020). In another study, Lovasi et al. (2009) found that the built environment impacted obesity in the community (Lovasi et al. 2009).[9] Obesity was associated with the lack of access to

---

[7] "To adjust for changes in the cost of living over time, historical income estimates in this report are expressed in real or 2021 dollars." The U.S. Census Bureau. https://www.census.gov/content/dam/Census/library/publications/2022/demo/p60-276.pdf.

[8] Researchers analyzed 2014 Medical Expenditure Panel (MEPS) Household Component Survey and the American Community Survey. The MEPS is a longitudinal study that collects U.S. family and individual data, including "demographic characteristics, health conditions, health status, use of medical services, charges and source of payments, access to care, satisfaction with care, health insurance coverage, income, and employment." U.S. Department of Health and Human Services. Agency for Healthcare and Research Quality. 2019. Medical Expenditure Panel Survey. https://www.meps.ahrq.gov/mepsweb/about_meps/survey_back.jsp. The American Community Survey is an annual survey that collects data on the U.S. population, including demographic, economic, and housing. U.S. States Census Bureau. https://www.census.gov/programs-surveys/acs.

[9] Obesity may lead to chronic health conditions such as type 2 diabetes, heart disease and stroke. Obesity is defined as a body mass index (BMI) equal to or greater than 30, and severe obesity is a BMI of 40 or greater. From 2017 to March 2020, Black adults (49.9%) had a higher prevalence of obesity than Hispanic adults (45.6%), White adults (41.4%), and Asian adults (16.1%). Based upon

healthy foods, exercise facilities, and community safety (Lovasi et al. 2009). The most disadvantaged groups lived in communities where the availability of healthy food, places to exercise, and safety was a challenge (Lovasi et al. 2009).

2.3 Algorithmic Bias as a Determinant of Health

The SDOH and algorithms may not seem to be interrelated, but they are. Similarly, algorithmic bias is a determinant of health because it affects where people live, work and play, much like SDOH. For example, financial institutions use algorithms to assess credit risk to make lending decisions (O'Neil 2016). These decisions can affect the neighborhood where people live, whether they purchase and/or rent a home, and their mode of transportation. Algorithms are used to screen job applications, determining if the person gets an interview, which may ultimately impact their economic stability (O'Neil 2016). Additionally, they impact how we "play" or socialize by determining what content is displayed on an individual's social media networks (O'Neil 2016). Algorithms also impact the school children attend, how people are evaluated academically and professionally, and the types of health services an individual may receive (Dans 2020; O'Neil 2016). This impact is magnified when the algorithms are biased. Algorithmic bias occurs when the algorithm is trained on data that are not diverse and representative. It can also occur when the algorithm measures the wrong outcome variable (Obermeyer et al. 2019; O'Neil 2016).

The algorithmic bias framework I propose is based upon the National Institute on Minority Health and Health Disparities (NIMHD) at NIH research framework (U.S. Department of Health and Human Services. National Institute on Minority Health and Health Disparities 2022). The NIMHD framework, published in 2019, is a multilevel model with multiple domains that conceptualize determinants that impact health (U.S. Department of Health and Human Services. National Institute on Minority Health and Health Disparities 2022). It "reflects an evolving conceptualization of factors relevant to the understanding and promotion of minority health and to the understanding and reduction of health disparities" (U.S. Department of Health and Human Services. National Institute on Minority Health and Health Disparities 2022). The framework builds upon the National Institute of Aging (NIA) health disparities research framework that focuses on environmental, sociocultural, behavioral, and biological domains as it relates to aging and health disparities (Hill et al. 2015). The NIMHD framework adopted the NIA model, renaming two of the domains (sociocultural environment and physical or built environment), adding the health care system domain, and categorizing the domains of determinants using the socioecological model (Alvidrez et al. 2019). The determinants are not meant to be

---

gender, Hispanic men (45.2%) were more obese than White men (43.1%), Black men (40.4%), and Asian men (17.6%). The prevalence of obesity in Black women (57.9%) was higher than Hispanic women (45.7%), White women (39.6%), and Asian women (14.5%), and all other groups. Black adults (14.0%) had the highest prevalence of of severe obesity than Hispanic adults (7.4%), White adults (9.5%), and Asian adults (1.8%) (Stierman et al. 2021).

		Levels of Influence			
		Individual	**Interpersonal**	**Community**	**Societal**
Domains of Influence	**Biological**	Biological Vulnerability and Mechanisms	Caregiver-Child Interaction Family Microbiome	Community Illness Exposure Herd Immunity	Sanitation Immunization Pathogen Exposure
	Behavioral	Health Behaviors Coping Strategies	Family Functioning School/Work Functioning	Community Functioning	Policies and Laws
	Physical/Built Environment	Personal Environment	Household Environment School/Work Environment	Community Environment Community Resources	Societal Structures
	Sociocultural Environment	Sociodemographics Limited English Cultural Identity Response to Discrimination	Social Networks Family/Peer Norms Interpersonal Discrimination	Community Norms Local Structural Discrimination	Social Norms Societal Structural Discrimination
	Health Care System	Insurance Coverage Health Literacy Treatment Preferences	Patient-Clinician Relationship Medical Decision-Making	Availability of Services Safety Net Services	Quality of Care Health Care Policies
	Algorithmic Bias	Employment Housing Access to Health Care and Health Services Education Economic	Social Networks Social media	Surveillance Resource Allocation	Data and Privacy Laws Regulation Equity
Health Outcomes		**Individual Health**	**Family/Organizational Health**	**Community Health**	**Population Health**

Fig. 2.2 Algorithmic bias framework: National Institute on Minority Health and Health Disparities expanded to include algorithmic bias

an exhaustive list. In the NIMHD framework, the SDOH are incorporated into the physical/built environment, sociocultural environment, and the health care system domains (Richardson et al. 2022). In this framework, algorithmic bias determinants are added to reflect their impact on health disparities (Fig. 2.2).

2.3.1 Individual-Level Determinants

At the individual level, algorithmic bias impacts employment, housing, access to health care and health services, education, and income (O'Neil 2016). For example, Amazon discovered that its recruitment algorithm under development, used for software engineer positions, was not gender neutral. The model was trained on historical 10-year-old data by observing patterns in resumes that were submitted (Dastin 2018; Köchling and Wehner 2020). During that timeframe, the resumes were mostly male applicants because they dominated the technology fields (Dastin 2018; Köchling and Wehner 2020). Thus, the model favored male over female candidates because most of the applicants in the tech field were male (Dastin 2018; Köchling and Wehner

2020). As a result, female candidates would be less likely to be recruited. The algorithmic tool was discontinued (Dastin 2018; Köchling and Wehner 2020).

Likewise, credit scores are thought to be race neutral. Under the Equal Credit Opportunity Act,[10] it is "unlawful for any creditor to discriminate against any applicant, with respect to any aspect of a credit transaction on the basis of race, color, religion, national origin, sex or marital status, or age (provided the applicant has the capacity to contract); because all or part of the applicant's income derives from any public assistance program; or because the applicant has in good faith exercised any right under this chapter." Credit worthiness determines if an individual can afford to rent or buy a home, purchase a car, can be approved for a credit card, can afford car insurance premiums, or qualify for a student loan (Singletary 2020). However, algorithms that determine creditworthiness may include or exclude factors that may disproportionately impact racial and ethnic minority populations (Singletary 2020). For example, rent payments are not usually included in credit score models. Additionally, the algorithms may rely on historical data reflective of discriminatory practices such as redlining[11] (Singletary 2020). This leads to unequal access to credit (Singletary 2020). Moreover, due to limited credit histories, the underlying data may be less accurate in predicting creditworthiness (Andrews 2021). Employment and creditworthiness impact where an individual works, his salary, where he can live, access to financial resources, and health.

2.3.2 Interpersonal-Level Determinants

Interpersonal-level determinants are an individual's connection and socialization with technology (Richardson et al. 2022). Algorithms impact how people connect socially. Previously, when Black girls, Asian girls, or Latina girls were inputted in Google's search engine algorithm, it would yield sexualized search results related to those populations (Noble 2018a, b). The prevalence of those type of results has subsequently decreased (Noble 2018a, b). In another example, when released in 2015, Google's photo app labeled pictures of Black people as gorillas (Grant and Hill 2023). In a *New York Times* article, the problem was attributed to the fact that the training data did not have enough images of Black people and confused darker-skinned Black people with gorillas (Grant and Hill 2023). Subsequently, Google has prevented its photo app from labeling anything a gorilla (Grant and Hill 2023).

There has also been concern that newsfeed algorithms on social media create political polarization by limiting a person's access to a wide range of content and instead providing more information from like-minded individuals who share similar

[10] Equal Credit Opportunity Act 15 15 U.S.C. 1691. https://www.govinfo.gov/content/pkg/USCODE-2011-title15/html/USCODE-2011-title15-chap41-subchapIV.htm.

[11] Redlining is "an illegal practice in which lenders avoid providing services to individuals living in communities of color because of the race or national origin of the people who live in those communities." U.S. Department of Justice. https://www.justice.gov/opa/pr/justice-department-announces-new-initiative-combat-redlining.

views, thus causing an echo chamber effect (Garcia 2023). Researchers found that downranking, or reducing the visibility, of all content from like-minded individuals, removing re-shared content, and disabling ranking calculations failed to reduce political polarization (Garcia 2023). However, down-ranking content and removing re-shares reduced misinformation and contact with untrustworthy sources (Garcia 2023).

Individuals who use social media may look for connection, information, or escapism. Depending upon the algorithm, they may face negative interactions, impacting their social and mental well-being. On the other hand, they may find linkages to groups and information that provide support and resources. However, if the algorithm is trained on biased data or is manipulative, it may impact the type of interactions the individual has with the technology.

2.3.3 Community Health-Level Determinants

Determinants at the community health level involve community well-being and the individual's feeling of security within the community. It embodies their interactions withing the community and the support that they receive. I suggest that this includes whether the systems in place within a community, be it local, state, or federal, are fair, just and equitable. For example, if an individual feels that they may be treated unjustly by the criminal justice system (i.e. an unlawful traffic stop, disproportionate sentencing) may be considered a community level determinant. As discussed in the previous chapter, Angwin et al. (2016) found that a risk assessment algorithm used to assess if a criminal defendant would likely re-offend found that Blacks were more likely to be incorrectly considered to have a higher recidivism risk than Whites (Angwin et al. 2016). The data used by the assessment tool did not include race; however, there were other data or proxy variables that could be associated with race (Angwin et al. 2016). In another example, Buolamwini and Gebru (2018) evaluated three commercial general classification systems and tested gender classification performance on darker-skinned females, darker-skinned males, lighter-skinned females, and lighter-skinned males (Buolamwini and Gebru 2018). They found dark-skinned females were the most misclassified group (Buolamwini and Gebru 2018). As facial recognition systems are being employed more for surveillance, an error can have detrimental real-world consequences for an individual that is wrongly misclassified (Buolamwini and Gebru 2018).

Lastly, Obermeyer et al. (2019) identified a racial bias in an algorithm used to predict the need for enrollment in health care management programs because the algorithm used health care costs as a proxy for health needs (Obermeyer et al. 2019). It appeared as though Whites needed additional health care services, despite the fact that Black patients were sicker (Obermeyer et al. 2019). What was not considered was that Blacks spent less on health care due to access barriers and discrimination, therefore using less health care management programs compared to Whites (Obermeyer et al. 2019). The source of the inaccuracy was identified as a labeling error (Obermeyer et al. 2019). The algorithm was subsequently fixed to prevent a future occurrence (Obermeyer et al. 2019).

2.3.4 *Societal-Level Determinants*

Societal-level determinants include laws, policies, and standards that regulate and impact algorithmic bias. For example, in 2023, over 25 U.S. states, Puerto Rico, and the District of Columbia introduced legislation regulating artificial intelligence (National Conference of State Legislators 2023). Examples include conducting a comprehensive inventory of all high-risk automated decision systems, minimizing the discriminatory impacts from automated decision systems, and quantifying the negative mental health risks associated with social media and AI (National Conference of State Legislators 2023). The U.S Federal Trade Commission (FTC), which indirectly regulates algorithms through its consumer protection authorities, filed a lawsuit against data brokers "for selling geolocation data from hundreds of millions of mobile devices that can be used to trace the movements of individuals to and from sensitive locations ... The FTC alleges that by selling data tracking people, [the company] is enabling others to identify individuals and exposing them to threats of stigma, stalking, discrimination, job loss, and even physical violence" (U.S. Federal Trade Commission 2022). The case was dismissed by the federal court because the FTC had not provided adequate evidence that there was substantial injury to the consumers but gave the agency an opportunity to strengthen its argument if they proceeded with the case (Singer 2023).

The White House Office of Science Policy and Technology, which will be discussed in Chapter Six, published the *Blueprint for an AI Bill of Rights* in 2022. It details five guiding principles in the design, use, and deployment of automated systems (The White House. Office of Science and Technology Policy 2022). They include safe and effective systems, algorithmic discrimination protections, data privacy, notice and explanation, and human alternatives, consideration, and fallback (The White House. Office of Science and Technology Policy 2022).

Laws, policies, and standards to regulate algorithmic bias serve to protect the public from their discriminatory impact. It is imperative that these safeguards exist to ensure health equity for racial and ethnic minority populations.

2.4 Summary

This chapter defined health disparities, discussed its economic impact, and examined its impact on racial and ethnic minority populations. The chapter also explained the social determinants of health—where people live, work, and play. Health disparities are complex. They are rooted in historical, biological, behavioral, environmental, socioeconomic, and cultural factors across the life course. They are also affected by the social determinants of health. Much like the social determinants of health, algorithmic bias also affects where people live, work, and play. If bias is embedded into the data, the algorithmic predictive ability will be compromised and can exacerbate disparities. Because their impact is so far-reaching, algorithmic bias is also a determinant of health.

References

Alvidrez, Jennifer, Dorothy Castille, Maryline Laude-Sharp, Adelaida Rosario, and Derrick Tabor. 2019. The National Institute on Minority Health and Health Disparities research framework. *American Journal of Public Health* 109 (Supp 1): S16–S20.

American Heart Association. 2016. What is high blood pressure? https://www.heart.org/en/health-topics/high-blood-pressure/the-facts-about-high-blood-pressure/what-is-high-blood-pressure. Accessed May 7, 2023.

Andrews, Edmund. 2021. *How flawed data aggravates inequality in credit.* Stanford University Human Centered Artificial Intelligence. https://hai.stanford.edu/news/how-flawed-data-aggravates-inequality-credit. Accessed August 20, 2023.

Angwin, Julia, Jeff Larson, Surya Mattu, and Lauren Kirchner. 2016. Machine bias. There's software used across the country to predict future criminals. And it's biased against blacks. *ProPublica.* https://www.propublica.org/article/machine-bias-risk-assessments-in-criminal-sentencing. Accessed August 20, 2023.

Arias, E., B. Tejada-Vera, K. Kochanek, and F.B. Ahmad. 2022. NVSS vital statistics rapid release: Provisional life expectancy estimates for 2021. https://www.cdc.gov/nchs/data/vsrr/vsrr023.pdf. Accessed September 19, 2023.

Buolamwini, J., and T. Gebru. 2018. Gender shades: Intersectional accuracy disparities in commercial gender classification. *Proceedings of Machine Learning Research* 81: 77–91.

Creamer, Johns, Emily A. Shrider, Kalee Burns, and Frances Chen. 2022. *Poverty in the United States: 2021.* U.S. Census Bureau, U.S. Government Publishing Office, Current Population Reports: 60-277. https://www.census.gov/content/dam/Census/library/publications/2022/demo/p60-277.pdf. Accessed September 20, 2023.

Cunningham, T.J., J.B. Croft, Y. Liu, H. Lu, P.I. Eke, and W.H. Giles. 2017. Vital signs: Racial disparities in age-specific mortality among blacks or African Americans—United States, 1999–2015. *MMWR. Morbidity and Mortality Weekly Report* 66: 444–456.

Dans, Enrique. 2020. Algorithms and education: Not so fast. *Forbes.* https://www.forbes.com/sites/enriquedans/2020/09/04/algorithms-and-education-not-sofast/?sh=71be1c1e446e. Accessed September 25, 2023.

Dastin, Jeffrey. 2018. Amazon scraps secret AI recruiting tool that showed bias against women. *Reuters.* https://www.reuters.com/article/us-amazon-com-jobs-automation-insight-idUSKCN1MK08G. Accessed August 20, 2023.

Ely, Danielle, and Anne K. Driscoll. 2020. Infant mortality in the United States, 2020: Data from the period linked birth/infant death file. *National Vital Statistics Reports* 71 (5).

Ely, Danielle M., and Donna L. Hoyert. 2018. Differences between rural and urban areas in mortality rates for the leading causes of infant death: United States, 2013–2015. *NCHS Data Brief* 300: 1–8.

Evans, Gary, and Pilyoung Kim. 2013. Childhood poverty, chronic stress, self-regulation and coping. *Child Development Perspectives* 7 (1): 43–48.

Forde, Allana T., Mario Sims, Paul Muntner, Tené Lewis, Amanda Onwuka, Kari Moore, and Ana V. Diez Roux. 2020. Discrimination and hypertension risk among African Americans in the Jackson Heart Study. *Hypertension* 76 (3): 715–723.

Garcia, David. 2023. Influence of Facebook algorithms on political polarizations tested. *Nature* 620: 39–41. https://doi.org/10.1038/d41586-023-02325-x.

Gracia, J. Nadine. 2018. Remembering Margaret Heckler's commitment to advancing minority health. *Health Affairs Blog*. https://www.healthaffairs.org/do/10.1377/hblog20181115.296624/full/. Accessed May 7, 2023.

Grant, Nico, and Kashmir Hill. 2023. Google's photo app still can't find gorillas. And neither can Apple's. *The New York Times*. https://www.nytimes.com/2023/05/22/technology/ai-photo-labels-google-apple.html. Accessed August 20, 2023.

Hill, Carl V., Eliseo J. Perez-Stable, Norman A. Anderson, and Marie A. Bernard. 2015. The national institute on aging health disparities research framework. *Ethnicity and Disease* 25 (3): 245–254. https://doi.org/10.18865/ed.25.3.245.

Institute of Medicine (U.S.) Committee on Understanding and Eliminating Racial and Ethnic Disparities in Health Care. 2003. *Unequal treatment: Confronting racial and ethnic disparities in health care*, ed. by B.D. Smedley, A.Y. Stith, and A.R. Nelson. Washington, DC: National Academies Press.

Karoly, Lynn A., M. Rebecca Kilburn, and Jill S. Cannon. 2005. *Early childhood interventions: Proven results, future promises*. Rand Corporation.

Keisler-Starkey, Katherine, and Lisa N. Bunch. 2022. *Health insurance coverage in the United States: 2021*. U.S. Census Bureau, U.S. Government Publishing Office, Current Population Reports: 60-278. https://www.census.gov/content/dam/Census/library/publications/2022/demo/p60-278.pdf. Accessed August 17, 2023.

Köchling, Alina, and Marius Claus Wehner. 2020. Discriminated by an algorithm: A systematic review of discrimination and fairness by algorithmic decision-making in the context of H.R. recruitment and H.R. development. *Business Research* 13: 795–848.

Lacour, Misty, and Laura D. Tissington. 2011. The effects of poverty on academic achievement. *Educational Research and Reviews* 6 (7): 522–527.

LaVeist, Thomas A., Darrel Gaskin, and Patrick Richard. 2011. Estimating the economic burden of racial health inequalities in the United States. *International Journal of Health Services* 41 (2): 231–238.

LaVeist, Thomas, Eliseo J. Pérez-Stable, Patrick Richard, Andrew Anderson, Lydia A. Isaac, Riley Santiago, Celine Okoh, Nancy Breen, Tilda Farhat, Assen Assenov, and Darrell J. Gaskin. 2023. The economic burden of racial, ethnic, and educational health inequities in the U.S. *JAMA* 329 (19): 1682–1692. https://doi.org/10.1001/jama.2023.5965.

Lovasi, Gina S., Malo A. Hutson, Monica Guerra, and Kathryn M. Neckerman. 2009. Built environments and obesity in disadvantaged populations. *Epidemiologic Reviews* 31: 7–20.

March of Dimes. 2022. Maternity care deserts report. Nowhere to go: Maternity care deserts across the U.S. https://www.marchofdimes.org/maternity-care-deserts-report. Accessed August 14, 2023.

National Conference of State Legislators. 2023. Legislation related to artificial intelligence. https://www.ncsl.org/technology-and-communication/artificial-intelligence-2023-legislation. Accessed June 24, 2023.

Noble, Sofiya Umoja. 2018a. *Algorithms of oppression: How search engines reinforce racism*. New York: NYU Press.

Noble, Sofiya Umoja. 2018b. Google has a striking history of bias against black girls. *Time*. https://time.com/5209144/google-search-engine-algorithm-bias-racism/. Accessed August 20, 2023.

Obermeyer, Ziad, Brian Powers, Christine Vogeli, and Sendhil Mullainathan. 2019. Dissecting racial bias in an algorithm used to manage the health of populations. *Science* 366: 447–453.

O'Neil, Cathy. 2016. *Weapons of math destruction*. New York: Broadway Books.

Ostchega, Yechiam, Cheryl D. Fryar, Tatiana Nwankwo, and Duong T. Nguyen. 2021. Hypertension prevalence among adults aged 18 and over: United States, 2017–2018. https://www.cdc.gov/nchs/data/databriefs/db364-h.pdf. Assessed September 17, 2023.

Pate, Cynthia A., Xiaoting Qin, Cathy M. Bailey, and Hatice S. Zahran. 2020. Cost barriers to asthma care by health insurance type among children with asthma. *Journal of Asthma* 57 (10): 1103–1109.

Richardson, Safiya, Katherine Lawrence, Antoinette M. Schoenthaler, and Devin Mann. 2022. A framework for digital health equity. *npj Digital Medicine* 5: 119. https://doi.org/10.1038/s41746-022-00663-0.

Semega, Jessica and Kollar, Melissa. 2022. Income in the United States: 2021. U.S. Census Bureau, U.S. Government Publishing Office, Current Population Reports: 60–276. https://www.census.gov/content/dam/Census/library/publications/2022/demo/p60-276.pdf. Assessed November 27, 2023.

Singer, Natasha. 2023. Judge dismisses F.T.C. lawsuit against a location data broker. *The New York Times*. https://www.nytimes.com/2023/05/05/business/ftc-kochava-location-data.html. Accessed August 20, 2023.

Singletary, Michelle. 2020. Credit scores are supposed to be race-neutral. That's impossible. *The Washington Post*. https://www.washingtonpost.com/business/2020/10/16/how-race-affects-your-credit-score/. Accessed August 20, 2023.

Smith, Genee S., Rachael R. McCleary, and Roland J. Thorpe, Jr. 2020. Racial disparities in hypertension prevalence within U.S. gentrifying neighborhoods. *International Journal of Environmental Research and Public Health* 17 (21): 7889.

Stierman, Bryan, Joseph Afful, Margaret D. Carroll, Te-Ching Chen, Orlando Davy, Steven Fink, Cheryl D. Fryar, Qiuping Gu, Craig M. Hales, Jeffery P. Hughes, Yechiam Ostchega, Renee J. Storandt, and Lara J. Akinbami. 2021. National Health and Nutrition Survey 2017-March 2020 Prepandemic Data Files-Development of Files and Prevalence Estimates for Selected Health Outcomes. National Health Statistics Reports; no 158. Hyattsville, MD: National Center for Health Statistics. 2021. https://dx.doi.org/10.15620/cdc:106273.

The White House. Office of Science and Technology Policy. 2022. Blueprint for an AI bill of rights. https://www.whitehouse.gov/ostp/ai-bill-of-rights/. Accessed July 24, 2023.

U.S. Department of Health and Human Services. Centers for Disease Control and Prevention. 2021. Social determinants of health at CDC. https://www.cdc.gov/socialdeterminants/about.html. Accessed May 8, 2023.

U.S. Department of Health and Human Services. Margaret M. Heckler. 1985. Report of the secretary's task force on black and minority health. https://ia600501.us.archive.org/32/items/reportofsecretar00usde/reportofsecretar00usde_bw.pdf. Accessed May 5, 2023.

U.S. Department of Health and Human Services. National Institutes of Health. 2021. Minority health and health disparities strategic plan 2021–2025. https://www.nimhd.nih.gov/docs/nimhd-strategic-plan-2021-2025.pdf. Accessed May 7, 2023.

U.S. Department of Health and Human Services. National Institutes of Health. 2023. Press release: NIH-funded study highlights the financial toll of health disparities in the United States. https://www.nih.gov/news-events/news-releases/nih-funded-study-highlights-financial-toll-health-disparities-united-states. Accessed August 14, 2023.

U.S. Department of Health and Human Services. National Institutes of Health. National Institute on Minority Health and Health Disparities. 2023. The economic burden of racial, ethnic, and educational health disparities in the U.S., 2018. https://www.nimhd.nih.gov/about/publications/economic-burden-health-disparities-US-2018.html. Accessed August 14, 2023.

U.S. Department of Health and Human Services. National Institute on Minority Health and Health Disparities. 2022. NIMHD research framework. https://www.nimhd.nih.gov/about/overview/research-framework/nimhd-framework.html. Accessed August 15, 2023.

U.S. Department of Health and Human Services. Office of the Assistant Secretary for Health. Office of Disease Prevention and Health Promotion. 2022. Health equity and health disparities environmental scan. https://health.gov/sites/default/files/2022-04/HP2030-HealthEquityEnvironmentalScan.pdf. Accessed August 17, 2023.

U.S. Federal Trade Commission. 2022. FTC sues Kochava for selling state that tracks people at reproductive health clinics, places of worship, and other sensitive locations. https://www.ftc.gov/news-events/news/press-releases/2022/08/ftc-sues-kochava-selling-data-tracks-people-reproductive-health-clinics-places-worship-other. Accessed August 20, 2023.

Whitehead, M. 1992. The concepts and principles of equity and health. *International Journal of Health Services* 22 (3): 429–445.

World Health Organization. 2018. Health inequities and their causes. https://www.who.int/news-room/facts-in-pictures/detail/health-inequities-and-their-causes. Accessed August 13, 2023.

World Health Organization. 2021. Social determinants of health. https://www.who.int/health-topics/social-determinants-of-health#tab=tab_1. Accessed June 8, 2021.

Zajacova, Anna, and Elizabeth M. Lawrence. 2018. The relationship between education and health: Reducing disparities through a contextual approach. *Annual Review of Public Health* 39: 273–289. https://www.ncbi.nlm.nih.gov/pmc/articles/PMC5880718/. Accessed August 14, 2023.

Chapter 3
The Inclusion of Racial and Ethnic Minority Groups in Clinical Trials

Abstract Clinical trials, also known as clinical studies, are research studies performed on people to evaluate the effectiveness and safety of a medical treatment, protocol, or device. The participation of racial and ethnic minority groups in clinical trials research is crucial to ensure data quality and generalizability. Most clinical trials lack adequate participation of racial and ethnic minority groups. One reason is mistrust due to a history of scientific research abuse. Section 3.1 discusses the changing demographics of the U.S. population. Section 3.2 defines clinical research and explores the lack of participation among racial and ethnic minority groups in clinical trials. Section 3.3 focuses on historical trauma and how past clinical abuses may contribute to mistrust in clinical trial participation. Section 3.4 summarizes key themes in this chapter.

Keywords Diversity · Clinical trials · Barriers to participation · Historical trauma · Mistrust · Data

3.1 Population Demographics in the United States

Race is a social construct, but it is used to classify people, quantify populations, allocate resources, and formulate public policy. As the United States becomes more racially and ethnically diverse, diversity in clinical research is urgently important and necessary (Vespa et al. 2020). According to the U.S. Census Bureau's July 2022 population estimates, Whites[1] comprised 75.5% of the U.S. population, followed by

[1] White is a person with origins in Europe, the Middle East, or North Africa. "It includes people who indicate their race as White or report Irish, German, Italian, German, Lebanese, Arab, Moroccan, or Caucasian." https://www.census.gov/topics/population/race/about.html.

N. H. Williams, *Artificial Intelligence and Healthcare*, The International Library of Bioethics 107, https://doi.org/10.1007/978-3-031-48262-5_3

Hispanics or Latinos (19.1%),[2] Blacks (13.6%),[3] Asians (6.3%),[4] Two or More Races (3.0%),[5] American Indians and Alaska Natives (1.3%),[6] and Native Hawaiians and Other Pacific Islanders (0.3%)[7] (U.S. Census Bureau 2023). Beginning in 2045, it is projected that most of the U.S. population will belong to a minority group (Vespa et al. 2020).[8] Thus, racial and ethnic minority groups will become the majority population when compared to Whites. By 2060, only 36.4% of children under 18 years old will be White. Moreover, by 2060, the number of immigrants living in the United States is projected to grow from 44 million in 2016 to 69 million (Vespa et al. 2020). This will reflect a growth from 14% to 17% of the U.S. population (Vespa et al. 2020). In short, by 2060, the U.S. population will be more racially and ethnically diverse, with population growth driven by immigration (Vespa et al. 2020). Whites will still be the largest race or ethnic group in the United States, but they will no longer be in the majority (Vespa et al. 2020).

Despite the current demographic composition of the United States, it is estimated that less than 10% of clinical trial participants were racial and ethnic minority groups (Vickers and Fouad 2014). It is estimated that only five percent of Blacks and one percent of Hispanics or Latinos were clinical trial participants nationally (The Society for Women's Health Research and the U.S. Food and Drug Administration Office of Women's Health 2011). In many instances, racial and ethnic minority groups suffer from higher rates of disease than their White counterparts. For example, in 2018, Blacks were "50 percent more likely to have a stroke" (U.S. Department of Health and Human Services, Office of Minority Health 2023); Asian Americans were nearly "eight times more likely to die from hepatitis B" (U.S. Department of Health and Human Services, Office of Minority Health 2020); American Indians/Alaska Natives were more than "50 percent likely to be diagnosed with coronary heart disease" (U.S. Department of Health and Human Services, Office of Minority Health 2021a); and Hispanics were "1.3 times more likely to die from diabetes" than Whites (U.S. Department of Health and Human Services, Office of Minority Health 2021b). Additionally, Native Hawaiians/Pacific Islanders' infant mortality rate was "almost

---

[2] Hispanic or Latino is a person of "Cuban, Mexican, Puerto Rican, South or Central American, or other Spanish culture or origin regardless of race." https://www.census.gov/topics/population/race/about.html.

[3] "Black or African American is a person with origins in any Black racial group of Africa." https://www.census.gov/topics/population/race/about.html.

[4] "Asian is a person with origins in the Far East, Southeast Asia, or the Indian subcontinent." https://www.census.gov/topics/population/race/about.html.

[5] "Two or More Races is the combination of two or more race categories." https://www.census.gov/topics/population/race/about.html.

[6] "American Indian and Alaska Native is a person with origins in North and South America (including Central America) and maintains tribal affiliation or community attachment." https://www.census.gov/topics/population/race/about.html.

[7] Native Hawaiian and Other Pacific Islander is "a person with origins in Hawaii, Guam, Samoa, or other Pacific Islands." https://www.census.gov/topics/population/race/about.html.

[8] "A minority group is categorized as Black or African American, American Indian and Alaska Native, Asian, and Native Hawaiian and Other Pacific Islander." https://www.census.gov/topics/population/race/about.html.

twice the infant mortality" as compared to Whites (U.S. Department of Health and Human Services, Office of Minority Health 2021c). Bearing in mind the impending demographic shift and the disparities in disease rates, representation of racial and ethnic minority groups in clinical research is critical. Diversity and inclusion are important in clinical trials because:

> People may experience the same disease differently. It's essential that clinical trials include people with a variety of lived experiences and living conditions, as well as characteristics like race and ethnicity, age, sex, and sexual orientation, so that all communities can benefit from scientific advances ... Historically, clinical trials did not always recruit participants who represented the individuals most affected by a particular disease, condition, or behavior. Often, these clinical trials relied almost exclusively on White male study participants. This shortcoming has created gaps in our understanding of diseases and conditions, preventive factors, and treatment effectiveness across populations. These gaps in knowledge can impede the quality of health care decision making, ability to counsel people on ways to reduce their risk, optimal treatment responses, and even the development of more effective medications or interventions. (U.S. Department of Health and Human Services, National Institute on Minority Health and Health Disparities, National Institutes of Health 2023)

3.2 What is Clinical Research and the Importance of Diversity in Participation

There are different types of clinical research. These include epidemiological,[9] behavioral,[10] health services,[11] and clinical trials[12] (U.S. Department of Health and Human Services, National Institutes of Health 2022). Clinical research differs from medical and clinical care because clinical research is for investigation and validation of interventions, whereas the former is for treatment and care (Eskew et al. 2013). In clinical research, the research objectives guide the study priorities, not the needs of the study participants (Eskew et al. 2013). The U.S. Food and Drug Administration (FDA) defines clinical research to include treatment research,[13] prevention

[9] Epidemiological research studies "the patterns, causes, and effects of the disease in specific populations." https://www.nih.gov/health-information/nih-clinical-research-trials-you/basics.

[10] Behavioral research studies human behavior and its impact on health and disease. https://www.nih.gov/health-information/nih-clinical-research-trials-you/basics.

[11] Health services research examines access to health services, their costs, and the impact of care on the patient. https://www.nih.gov/health-information/nih-clinical-research-trials-you/basics.

[12] Clinical trials evaluate the impact of a health intervention. https://www.nih.gov/health-information/nih-clinical-research-trials-you/basics.

[13] Treatment research "involves an intervention such as medication, psychotherapy, new devices, or new approaches to surgery or radiation therapy." https://www.fda.gov/patients/clinical-trials-what-patients-need-know/what-are-different-types-clinical-research.

research,[14] diagnostic research,[15] screening research,[16] quality of life research,[17] genetic studies,[18] as well as epidemiological studies and clinical trials (U.S. Food and Drug Administration 2018).

Both NIH and FDA describe clinical trials, also known as clinical studies, as research studies performed on people to evaluate the effectiveness and safety of a medical treatment, protocol, or device (U.S. Department of Health and Human Services, National Institutes of Health 2022; U.S. Food and Drug Administration 2020). The treatment can be a drug, gene therapy, vaccine, or a medical device (U.S. Department of Health and Human Services, National Institutes of Health 2022; U.S. Food and Drug Administration 2020). In the United States, clinical trials occur in four phases (Piña and Pines 2014; U.S. Food and Drug Administration 2018). In Phase I, the experimental drug or treatment is tested in a small group of people (approximately 20–80) to determine metabolic and pharmacological actions, side effects, appropriate dosage, and safety (Piña and Pines 2014; U.S. Food and Drug Administration 2018). During Phase II, the experimental drug or treatment is given to a larger group of people (up to several hundred) to determine safety, effectiveness, and confirm preliminary dosage data (Piña and Pines 2014; U.S. Food and Drug Administration 2018). In Phase III, the experimental drug or treatment is given to several thousand people to collect data to meet FDA approval, confirm effectiveness, and compare to other treatments (Piña and Pines 2014; U.S. Food and Drug Administration 2018). Finally, Phase IV trials occur after the drug or treatment is approved to monitor for adverse effects and other benefits (Piña and Pines 2014; U.S. Food and Drug Administration 2018). Clinical trials are voluntary, and the collected data determine whether the new pharmaceutical, treatment, or device is effective and safe for use. These data are extrapolated from the test population to the general population (Piña and Pines 2014; U.S. Food and Drug Administration 2018).

The data gained from clinical trial participation inform treatment protocols, lead to new methods of treating disease, and determine which interventions may be the most effective in specific populations (U.S. Department of Health and Human Services, National Institutes of Health 2022). However, the underreporting of race and ethnic

---

[14] Prevention research "looks for better ways to prevent disorders from developing or returning. For example, different kinds of prevention research may study medicines, vitamins, vaccines, minerals, or lifestyle changes." https://www.fda.gov/patients/clinical-trials-what-patients-need-know/what-are-different-types-clinical-research.

[15] Diagnostic research "refers to the practice of looking for better ways to identify a particular disorder or condition." https://www.fda.gov/patients/clinical-trials-what-patients-need-know/what-are-different-types-clinical-research.

[16] Screening research "aims to find the best ways to detect certain disorders or health conditions." https://www.fda.gov/patients/clinical-trials-what-patients-need-know/what-are-different-types-clinical-research.

[17] Quality of life research "explores ways to improve comfort and the quality of life for individuals with a chronic illness." https://www.fda.gov/patients/clinical-trials-what-patients-need-know/what-are-different-types-clinical-research.

[18] Genetic studies "aim to improve the prediction of disorders by identifying and understanding how genes and illnesses may be related." https://www.fda.gov/patients/clinical-trials-what-patients-need-know/what-are-different-types-clinical-research.

subgroup analysis is common, especially for Blacks and Hispanics (Khalil et al. 2022; Loree et al. 2019). The failure to enroll adequate numbers of racial and ethnic minority groups in clinical trials not only limits the generalizability of the results, but it may also overlook ethnic and racial differences in treatment response. Additionally, this failure prevents the identification of the positive and negative effects of the treatment in these populations, potentially leading to ineffective and deleterious impacts (Branson et al. 2007). Consequently, the clinical trial participant pool does not reflect the wider population where the treatment may be given. A drug may be effective in one population but deadly in another due to such factors as genetic variants (Oh et al. 2015). For instance, researchers discovered that Pacific Islanders could not convert a particular antiplatelet drug into an active form, thereby placing them at higher risk for complications following angioplasty (Mega et al. 2010; Oh et al. 2015). In another example, certain genetic variants (G1 and G2) of the plasma protein apolipoprotein L1 (APOL1) are associated with kidney disease in people of African descent but not in those of European ancestry (Friedman and Pollak 2016). These variants not only provide immunity to trypanosomiasis[19] but are also associated with chronic kidney disease in this population (Genovese et al. 2010; Limou et al. 2014; Parsa et al. 2013).

The recruitment and retention of individuals, especially racial and ethnic minorities, into clinical trials are paramount. However, research shows that both recruitment into clinical trials and high recidivism rates prove to be challenging among minority and low-income populations (Barnett et al. 2012; Branson et al. 2007). Low participation numbers in clinical trials may impact data validity and reliability due to diminished study power,[20] bias, and study generalizability (Branson et al. 2007). These are amplified with an underrepresentation of racial and ethnic minority groups. The underrepresentation limits the efficacy and safety generalizability to the larger population (Boden-Albala et al. 2015) (Fig. 3.1).

There are many reasons for low participation of racial and ethnic minority groups in clinical trials. Many are related to structural and systemic barriers that limit access. Examples include the lack of a recruitment infrastructure to enlist racial and ethnic minority populations, the underinsurance or lack of insurance of potential participants, restrictive clinical trial enrollment criteria that exclude potential participants, and the lack of clinical trials at under-resourced hospitals where racial and ethnic minorities may receive care (Boden-Albala et al. 2015). Other reasons are socioeconomic barriers for potential participants, including lack of transportation, time commitment away from work, and inflexible work schedules. Other causes are information-based, such as lack of physician knowledge about clinical trials, the absence of physician referrals, and the patients' lack of awareness of the clinical trials themselves and how to enroll (Boden-Albala et al. 2015; Hamel et al. 2016). Lastly,

[19] Trypanosomiasis, otherwise known as sleeping sickness, is fatal if not treated with medication. Some symptoms include headache, weakness, fatigue, weight loss, and intermittent fevers.

[20] Power is the ability of a statistical test to detect an effect in a population.

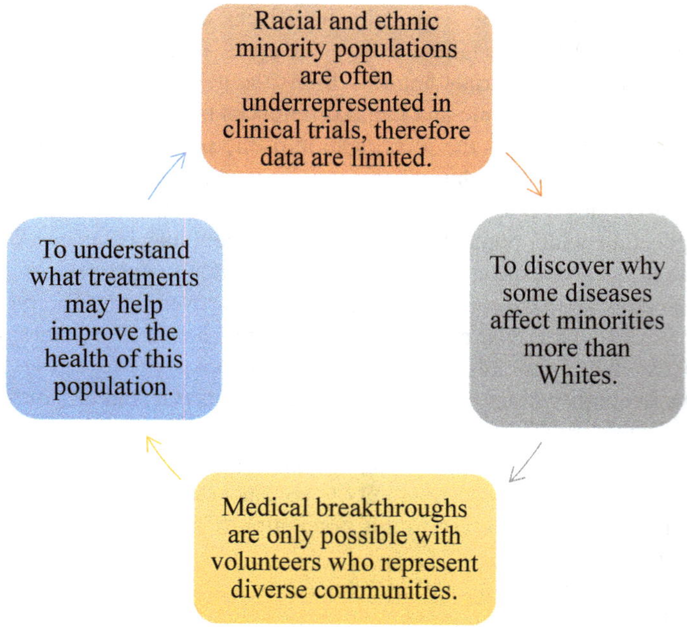

Fig. 3.1 The importance of racial and ethnic minority participation in clinical trials

sometimes clinical trial participation may depend upon whether the participant feels respected and valued in the process. Possible incentives to increase participation include access to medical care, medication, and medical information (Boden-Albala et al. 2015) (Fig. 3.2).

The most subtle barriers are potential participants' distrust of the medical provider and medical institutions, fear of experimentation and treatment side effects, and implicit and explicit bias, which may affect the referral process to clinical trials (Boden-Albala et al. 2015; Hamel et al. 2016). Most notably, they fear being exploited and mistreated. However, some research indicates that racial and ethnic minorities are just as willing to participate in clinical trials as Whites, but they are not asked to do so (Wendler et al. 2006). The willingness to participate arises from an altruistic desire to help those in their community, find a cure or treatment for the disease in question, and join for the greater good (Hughes et al. 2017). For example, this altruism was evident in news stories on the SARS-CoV-2 (COVID-19) vaccine clinical trials focused on minority participation and vaccine hesitancy. Those interviewed stated that their participation was for the greater good of the community or to set an example for others (Berg 2020; Turner and Wenger 2020).

Despite attempts to diversify participation in the COVID-19 vaccine clinical trials and to educate the public about the effectiveness of the vaccines through public health outreach campaigns, community engagement, and logistical support, many people remained suspicious of the vaccine. Some were concerned about the speed at which the vaccine was developed. Still others were misinformed about the vaccine's possible

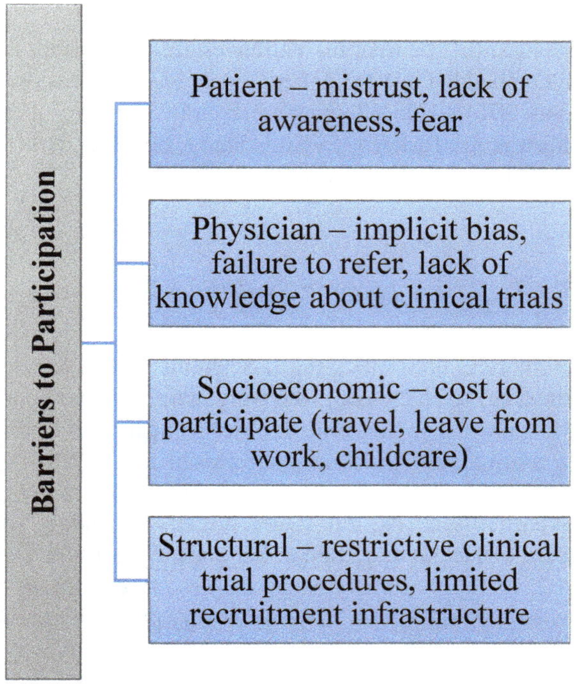

Fig. 3.2 Examples of barriers to clinical trial participation

side effects. In addition, access barriers prevented those who wanted to be vaccinated from receiving the vaccine. These barriers continue to be transportation challenges, language accessibility, computer illiteracy, and lack of internet access to schedule vaccine appointments (Lewis 2021; Luebbert and Perez 2016; Rubin 2014).

3.3 Historical Trauma

Despite the possible benefits of clinical trial participation, many racial and ethnic minority groups are circumspect to participate. The distrust stems from documented abuses in medical research. Historical trauma is "multigenerational trauma experienced by a specific cultural, racial or ethnic group. It is related to major events that oppressed a particular group of people because of their status as oppressed, such as slavery, the Holocaust, forced migration, and the violent colonization of Native Americans" (U.S. Department of Health and Human Services, Administration for Children and Families n.d.). In short, historical trauma is a trauma that is shared by a group that spans generations (Akinyemi 2022; Sacks et al. 2021; Sotero 2006; U.S. Department of Health and Human Services, Administration for Children and Families n.d.). Some may argue that such research atrocities happened decades ago, the potential participants were not alive when they happened, or that safeguards have been put in place to prevent future abuses (Berkowitz 2017; Mohatt et al. 2014). While these reasons may be true, the narratives are still shared, and the exploitation and abuse are embedded into the generational consciousness as a communal memory (Mohatt et al. 2014). The following are examples of clinical research abuses that perpetuate this trauma: Tuskegee Syphilis Study; Mrs. Henrietta Lacks; the Guatemala Syphilis Experiment; and Holmesburg Prison.

3.3.1 The Tuskegee Syphilis Study

From 1932 until 1972, the U.S. Public Health Service (USPHS) studied poor and uneducated Black men, who were mainly sharecroppers and tenant farmers in rural Macon County, Alabama, to observe the natural history of untreated, latent syphilis (Berkowitz 2017; Brandt 1978; Mohatt et al. 2014). Syphilis is a sexually transmitted disease (STD) that causes ulcerative lesions in the genitals, rectum, or mouth. Syphilis disease has four stages: primary, secondary, latent, and tertiary (U.S. Department of Health and Human Services, Centers for Disease Control and Prevention 2022a). In the primary stage, painless sores form at the spot of infection that heal within several weeks. In the secondary phase, symptoms may include lesions, fever, swollen lymph nodes, hair loss, weight loss, and fatigue (U.S. Department of Health and Human Services, Centers for Disease Control and Prevention 2022a). Sores may appear in the mouth or genital area. This phase may resolve within several weeks but may reappear up to a year later (U.S. Department of Health and Human Services, Centers for Disease Control and Prevention 2022a). The latent stage is asymptomatic and can last for years (U.S. Department of Health and Human Services, Centers for Disease Control and Prevention 2022a). When untreated, syphilis may progress to the tertiary phase, resulting in the impairment of the cardiovascular and central nervous systems and damage to vital organs, leading to dementia, paralysis, blindness, and death (U.S. Department of Health and Human Services, Centers for Disease Control and Prevention 2022a). Additionally, women with syphilis can spread the disease to their unborn children (U.S. Department of Health and Human Services, Centers for Disease Control and Prevention 2023a). Untreated congenital syphilis can cause premature birth, stillbirth, or death (U.S. Department of Health and Human Services, Centers for Disease Control and Prevention 2023a). In newborns, congenital syphilis can cause jaundice, anemia, deformed bones, deafness, and blindness (U.S. Department of Health and Human Services, Centers for Disease Control and Prevention 2023a).

In 1932, the USPHS researchers enrolled 399 men with latent syphilis and 201 men without syphilis to study the natural progression of the disease (U.S. Department of Health and Human Services, Centers for Disease Control and Prevention 2022b). The men who did not have syphilis served as the control group. However, when some of the men in the control group developed syphilis, they were switched to the syphilitic group (Williams 2008). Researchers told study participants that they were being treated for "bad blood" (U.S. Department of Health and Human Services, Centers for Disease Control and Prevention 2022b, 2023b). "Bad blood" was a phrase used to describe various conditions such as syphilis, amenia, muscle aches, and fatigue (Tuskegee University 2023; Williams 2008). However, there was no intention of treating the men's syphilis, even though penicillin was discovered as an effective treatment in 1947 (U.S. Department of Health and Human Services, Centers for Disease Control and Prevention 2023b; Williams 2008). Instead, the researchers provided ineffective treatments like aspirin, vitamins, arsenic, and mercury salve (U.S. Department of Health and Human Services, Centers for Disease Control and Prevention 2023b). In exchange for their participation, study participants were offered medical care, survivors' insurance, meals, transportation to and from the medical clinic, and burial expenses if they allowed an autopsy to be performed (U.S. Department of Health and Human Services, Centers for Disease Control and Prevention 2023b; Williams 2008). It was not until 1972 that the surviving study participants were told they had syphilis. Initially, this clinical study was projected to last only six months, but it lasted approximately 40 years (U.S. Department of Health and Human Services, Centers for Disease Control and Prevention 2023b; Williams 2008).

On July 25, 1972, the Associated Press reported that rural Black men were untreated for syphilis for 40 years as participants in a federal government research study (Heller 2017). As a result, in August 1972, the U.S. Department of Health, Education, and Welfare (HEW) (now known as the U.S. Department of Health and Human Services) appointed an advisory panel to investigate the Tuskegee Syphilis Study. The Tuskegee Syphilis Study Ad Hoc Advisory Panel (Advisory Panel) found that the study was unethical, scientifically unsound, and lacked a written protocol (U.S. Department of Health, Education, and Welfare, Public Health Service 1973). During its investigation into the circumstances of the study, the Advisory Panel discovered that there was no written protocol to the original study or documentation of the study's purpose. Inferring from direct statements, the Advisory Panel determined that the purpose of the study was:

> a) to study the natural history of disease; b) study the course of treated and untreated syphilis; c) study the differences in histological and clinical course of the disease in black versus white subjects; d) study with an "acceptance" of the postulate that there was a benign course of the disease in later stages vis-à-vis the dangers of available therapy; e) short-term study (6 months or longer) of the incidence and clinical course of late latent syphilis in the Negro male; and f) a study which would provide valuable data for a syphilis control program for a rural impoverished community. (U.S. Department of Health, Education, and Welfare, Public Health Service 1973, p. 6)

As stated by the Advisory Panel, not only were there no written study protocols, but there was also no evidence of informed consent, which was not analogous to voluntary participation (U.S. Department of Health, Education, and Welfare, Public Health Service 1973).

The Advisory Panel described the elements of informed consent. It included a description of the procedures, including those that are experimental; an explanation of the risks and benefits; disclosure of alternative treatments that may be beneficial; the offer to answer any questions about the study; and the ability of the participant to withdraw consent and participation in the study (U.S. Department of Health, Education, and Welfare, Public Health Service 1973). In addition, informed consent would have made the participants aware of the potential risk to themselves and the possible infection of others who were non-study participants, such as family and friends (U.S. Department of Health, Education, and Welfare, Public Health Service 1973). The Advisory Panel also found that the study lacked standardization of scientific procedures, which impacted study validity and reliability (U.S. Department of Health, Education, and Welfare, Public Health Service 1973). Moreover, the Advisory Panel concluded that penicillin therapy should have been provided to the program participants no later than 1953 when it became widely available (U.S. Department of Health, Education, and Welfare, Public Health Service 1973).

The Advisory Panel also reviewed a series of letters from February 1941 to August 1942 between study officials and local health officials (U.S. Department of Health, Education, and Welfare, Public Health Service 1973). Study participants under the age of 45 were drafted for army service but rejected because they were positive for syphilis. Consequently, study officials provided the local selective service board a list of 256 men under the age of 45 "asking that they be excluded from the list of draftees needing treatment" (U.S. Department of Health, Education, and Welfare, Public Health Service 1973, p. 10). The local selective service board complied, and the study continued. The men had already received notification by the local selective service boards to begin medical treatment for syphilis. According to Wenger, "the patients in the study received no treatment on our recommendation. At the present, we know that most of the participants in this study received some form of treatment with heavy metals and/or antibiotics. Although the adequacy of the treatment received is not known, it is clear that the treatment received was provided by physicians who were not part of the study and who were individually sought by the individual patients related to their own medical symptoms and pursuit of treatment" (U.S. Department of Health, Education, and Welfare, Public Health Service 1973, p. 10).

The Advisory Panel concluded that "the scientific merits of the Tuskegee Study are vastly overshadowed by the violation of basic ethic principles pertaining to human dignity and human life imposed on the experimental subjects" (U.S. Department of Health, Education, and Welfare, Public Health Service 1973, p. 11). The Tuskegee Study of Untreated Syphilis in the Negro Male officially ended in 1972, one month after the Advisory Panel recommended ending the study (U.S. Department of Health and Human Services, Centers for Disease Control and Prevention 2022b). The study participants and their families received a $10 million settlement after the 1973 class-action lawsuit filed against the U.S. government on their behalf was settled out of court (U.S. Department of Health and Human Services, Centers for Disease Control and Prevention 2023c). The settlement was divided into four categories. Living participants with syphilis received $37,500; the heirs of the deceased study participants with syphilis received $15,000; the "living control group participants received $16,000"; and the heirs of deceased study participants from the control group received $5000 (U.S. Department of Health and Human Services, Centers for Disease Control and Prevention 2023c).

The Tuskegee Health Benefit Program was established to administer lifetime medical benefits and burial services to the living participants who were also part of the settlement, which was expanded in 1975 to include the wives, widows, and children of the study participants. In 1995, the program expanded to include health and medical benefits (U.S. Department of Health and Human Services, Centers for Disease Control and Prevention 2022b). On May 16, 1997, President Bill Clinton issued an apology to the remaining survivors of the Syphilis Study at Tuskegee, stating in part:

> So today America does remember the hundreds of men used in research without their knowledge and consent. We remember them and their family members. Men who were poor and Black, without resources and with few alternatives, they believed they had found hope when they were offered free medical care by the United States Public Health Service. They were betrayed.
>
> Medical people are supposed to help when we need care, but even once a cure was discovered, they were denied help, and they were lied to by their government. Our government is supposed to protect the rights of its citizens; their rights were trampled upon. Forty years, hundreds of men betrayed, along with their wives and children, along with the community in Macon County, Alabama, the City of Tuskegee, the fine university there, and the larger African American community.
>
> The United States government did something that was wrong—deeply, profoundly, morally wrong. It was an outrage to our commitment to integrity and equality for all our citizens. (The White House, Office of the Press Secretary 1997)

When asked about the impact of the Tuskegee Study on minority participation in clinical studies during a 2002 discussion, the then U.S. Secretary of the Department of Health and Human Services responded that the study had a deleterious impact on African Americans' trust in the health care system (Sullivan 2002). Many questioned would they be subjected to experimentation or receive premium treatment (Sullivan 2002). Compounded by other negative interactions that African Americans have experienced with the health care system, there is a general distrust of medical professionals. This distrust has made it challenging to enroll African Americans in clinical trials (Sullivan 2002).

3.3.2 Mrs. Henrietta Lacks

In 1951, Mrs. Henrietta Lacks, a poor Black woman and mother of five was diagnosed with an aggressive form of cervical cancer at the Johns Hopkins Hospital in Baltimore, Maryland (Jennings 2017; Rao 2016; Skloot 2010). For diagnosis and treatment, her physician took a biopsy of the cancerous tissue. Without Mrs. Lacks' consent, a biopsy tissue sample was sent to a virologist and cancer researcher who collected cancer cell samples and grew them in his lab (Rao 2016). While other cell samples perished, Mrs. Lacks' cells continued to grow (Rao 2016). Mrs. Lacks died from cervical cancer within the same year of her diagnosis at the age of 31 (Jennings 2017; Rao 2016).

Later, known as HeLa cells, these cells were the first human cell line that continuously reproduced without dying (Skloot 2010). As a result, they were foundational in scientific research and medical advances such as the polio vaccine, immunology, genomics, and cancer research (Johns Hopkins Medicine n.d.). However, during Mrs. Lacks' biopsy, no consent was required for the removal of her cells; therefore, neither Mrs. Lacks nor her family granted permission or were compensated for their use (Johns Hopkins Medicine n.d.). Her family was unaware of their use until 1973 (McKie 2010). In 2013, the Johns Hopkins Hospital, National Institutes of Health, and the Lacks family established an agreement that required researchers to obtain permission for their use (Hudson and Collins 2013). Johns Hopkins did not sell or profit from the cell lines. However, the agreement did not provide the Lacks family with any financial proceeds from research on the HeLa genome (Zimmer 2013). In 2021, the Lacks family filed a federal lawsuit against the biotechnology company Thermo Fisher Scientific, arguing that they used her cells without consent (Gamble 2023; Skene and Brumfield 2023). They contended that even after the origin of the cells became known, the company still commercialized their use and received substantial financial benefit from it (Gamble 2023; Skene and Brumfield 2023). There was a confidential out-of-court settlement between her family and the biotechnology company in August 2023 (Gamble 2023; Skene and Brumfield 2023).

The case of Mrs. Henrietta Lacks occurred before the establishment of the U.S. Federal Policy for the Protection of Human Subjects in 1991, otherwise known as the Common Rule (Williams 2005). It was initially published in 1974 and revised throughout the years, most recently in 2018 (U.S. Department of Health and Human Services, Office for Human Research Protections 2023; Williams 2005). The Common Rule governs most federally funded research in the United States, providing for the protection of human research subjects (Williams 2005). It outlines the extensive requirements for informed consent, the review of proposed research by an Institutional Review Board, and compliance with federal research requirements (Williams 2005).

3.3.3 The Guatemala Syphilis Experiment

The Guatemala Syphilis Experiment is another example of historical research abuse. The research focused on the transmission and treatment of syphilis, gonorrhea, and chancroid, as well as serological diagnostic testing (Presidential Commission for the Study of Bioethical Issues 2011). Between 1946 and 1948, USPHS researchers, with the aid of the Guatemalan government, intentionally infected at least 1308 prisoners, soldiers, and psychiatric patients with syphilis, gonorrhea, and chancroid without their knowledge or consent, to study disease transmission and treatment (Presidential Commission for the Study of Bioethical Issues 2011; Rodriguez and Garcia 2013). Through 1953, approximately 5100 study participants, including children, mental health patients, soldiers, prisoners, and leprosy patients, were subjected to serological diagnostic tests that included lumbar[21] and cisternal[22] punctures (Rodriguez and Garcia 2013). In November 1946, researchers began to test prison inmates, psychiatric hospital patients, and leprosy patients, identifying those with syphilis (Presidential Commission for the Study of Bioethical Issues 2011). The purpose was to validate the serological testing and ensure a reliable diagnosis of syphilis. The lumbar punctures were done on some subjects to confirm the serological blood test results (Presidential Commission for the Study of Bioethical Issues 2011). Of the thousands tested for STDs, there were 842 inmates, 51 leprosy patients, and 642 psychiatric patients (Presidential Commission for the Study of Bioethical Issues 2011). From 1947 to 1949, the researchers expanded their test population to include children. They tested over 1300 Guatemalan children from ages one to 18 for STDs (Presidential Commission for the Study of Bioethical Issues 2011). These children were from orphanages, rural communities, and state-run schools. The children were not inoculated or exposed to an STD during this stage (Presidential Commission for the Study of Bioethical Issues 2011). The rationale for testing children who were not pubescent was "to ensure the opportunity for conclusive evidence of false positivity for any testing regime, because subjects presumably would have acquired the disease congenitally rather than sexually, and congenital syphilis was distinguishable" (Presidential Commission for the Study of Bioethical Issues 2011, p. 38). The children were unaware that they were experimental participants, and there was no record of consent given by their parents or guardians (Presidential Commission for the Study of Bioethical Issues 2011). Not only were the children subjected to blood tests, but many underwent physical exams, which included the examination of genitalia for males. Some children also endured lumbar punctures (Presidential Commission for the Study of Bioethical Issues 2011).

During the exposure experiments, approximately 1300 people ranging from ages 10 to 72 were intentionally exposed to gonorrhea, syphilis, and chancroid (Presidential Commission for the Study of Bioethical Issues 2011). Those included were Guatemalan soldiers, prisoners, psychiatric patients, and sex workers. Of this number, nearly 700 received treatment. Methods of exposure depended upon the STD. For gonorrhea, exposure included sexual contact, penile inoculation, cervical inoculation after sexual contact, and inoculation of the rectum, urethra, and eyes. For the syphilis experiments, people were exposed through sexual contact, digestion, injection with syphilitic material, and cisternal puncture. The researchers exposed subjects by cutaneous inoculation in the chancroid experiments (Presidential Commission for the Study of Bioethical Issues 2011).

On October 1, 2010, President Barack Obama apologized to Guatemalan President Alvaro Colom and the people of Guatemala for the medical research. Along with Kathleen Sebelius, Secretary of the U.S. DHHS, and Hillary Rodham Clinton, Secretary of the Department of State, he issued a joint apology to the government

[21] A lumbar puncture is the insertion of a needle between two lumbar vertebrae to remove the spinal fluid.

[22] A cisternal puncture is the insertion of a needle into the back of the skull into the spinal fluid.

of Guatemala (Presidential Commission for the Study of Bioethical Issues 2011). On November 24, 2010, President Obama appointed the Presidential Commission for the Study of Bioethical Issues (Commission) to investigate the Guatemala study and to review federal and international human subject protections to ensure that they safeguard participants in scientific studies (Presidential Commission for the Study of Bioethical Issues 2011).

With its mandate from the President, the Commission studied: (1) what happened in Guatemala during the USPHS-funded study; (2) the awareness and enforcement of the research protocols by the federal officials and other medical researchers; (3) the historical context of the studies and research ethics at that time, and (4) whether there was a deviation from those ethical standards (Presidential Commission for the Study of Bioethical Issues 2011). Issuing its report in September 2011, the Commission found that consent was not obtained from the research subjects; the experimental design and its execution were unorganized; the risks and benefits were not told to the research subjects; and it preyed on the most vulnerable in society (Presidential Commission for the Study of Bioethical Issues 2011). In conclusion, the Commission determined:

> As a direct result of the decisions and actions of the PHS researchers and their superiors, profoundly vulnerable persons, some in the saddest and most despairing states, had their bodies systematically and repeatedly violated. An intense and uncritical commitment to advancing knowledge under convenient conditions does not account for the suspension of moral sensitivity that should have been stimulated by the suffering of their fellow persons, suffering that the researchers themselves, in some cases, grievously aggravated. It is clear that many of the actions undertaken within the Guatemala experiments were morally wrong. The Commission further concludes that the individuals who approved, conducted, facilitated, and funded these experiments are morally culpable to various degrees for these wrongs. (Presidential Commission for the Study of Bioethical Issues 2011, p. 108)

3.3.4 Holmesburg Prison

One of the most notorious cases of prisoner abuse occurred at the Holmesburg Prison in Pennsylvania. Allen M. Hornblum's book, *Acres of Skin: Human Experiments at Holmesburg Prison; A True Story of Abuse and Exploitation in the Name of Medicine,* recounted abuses at the Holmesburg Prison in Philadelphia by Dr. Albert Kligman, a dermatologist at the University of Pennsylvania (Hornblum 1998). Between 1951 and 1974, prison inmates were subjected to tests involving various consumer products, including shampoo, deodorant, skin creams, eye drops, diet drinks, hair dyes, and detergents, which were followed by skin biopsies and exploratory experiments (Goodman 1998; Hornblum 1998). In exchange, inmates were paid $10 to $300 compared with the prison wages of 15 cents or 25 cents a day. Often, the inmates were poor, Black, uneducated, and ill-informed about the testing (Goodman 1998).

In one 1972 study, shampoo was dropped into the eyes of 20 prisoners for 24 hours. The inmates only received $3.00 each (U.S. Senate Hearings 1973). Mind-altering drugs and dioxin were tested on the inmates, too (Goodman 1998; Robbins 1993).

The dioxin tests exposed inmates to the most potent form of dioxin called 2,3,7,8-tetrachlorodibenzo-p-dioxin (TCDD) (Robbins 1993; U.S. Department of Health and Human Services 2018). During the 1960s, TCDD was used as a pesticide and as Agent Orange (herbicide defoliator) during the Vietnam War (Robbins 1993; U.S. Senate Hearings 1973). Despite being warned that TCDD was highly toxic, Dr. Kligman increased the administered dosage from 16 to 7500 μg after the initial test group failed to show any symptoms (Robbins 1993). The inmates developed lesions, some of which became inflamed pustules that lasted several months (Robbins 1993).

In her book, *Medical Apartheid: The Dark History of Medical Experimentation on Black Americans from Colonial Times to the Present,* Harriet A. Washington detailed the horror these prisoners endured at Holmesburg Prison (Williams 2008). One inmate described radiation and sulfuric acid burns, chemicals being rubbed on his scrotum, removal of skin, implantation of cadaver tissue into his back, chemical patch tests, and slashes under his arms to study his lymph nodes, among other disfiguring experiments (Williams 2008). Washington wrote that prisoners were also injected with herpes, syphilis, gonorrhea, and malaria. Many inmates suffered lingering effects from the experimentation, including skin disfiguration and cancers (Williams 2008).

Prisoner experimentation was not limited solely to Holmesburg Prison; it also occurred in other locations in the Philadelphia County Prisons (U.S. Senate Hearings 1973). In 1973, during the U.S. Senate Hearings before the Subcommittee on Health of the Committee on Labor and Public Welfare, when asked if there were informed consent waivers, the witness replied, "You have informed consent waivers, but that, to more of the men in a penitentiary, is like reading hieroglyphics" (U.S. Senate Hearings 1973, p. 825). Witnesses testified that "many of the prisoners, who were poor, became involved in the experiments because they needed to raise money for bail, provide for families, hire attorneys, and purchase basic necessities" (U.S. Senate Hearings 1973, p. 825).

3.4 Summary

The population demographics in the United States are changing. As the population becomes more diverse, clinical research must reflect the diversity in society. Diversity ensures that medical discoveries are available for all people, not just for those who meet an outdated gender and racial paradigm. There are many reasons for the lack of participation in clinical research among racial and ethnic minority groups such as clinical trial barriers, health care providers' lack of awareness, the lack of access to clinical trials, socioeconomic factors, not feeling respected and valued during the process, and mistrust. This mistrust is borne from the historical trauma resulting from medical abuse and experimentation.

The failure to enroll adequate numbers of racial and ethnic minority groups in clinical research not only constrains the generalizability of the results, but it may overlook ethnic and racial differences in treatment response. As discussed in earlier chapters, if racial and ethnic minority groups are not adequately represented or missing from data that are used to train algorithmic models in general, this may create biased predictions, reduced accuracy, and limited generalizability. Therefore, it is paramount that that racial and ethnic minorities are included in clinical research.

References

Akinyemi, Adebisi. 2022. Historical trauma compounds experiences of racial injustice. *Nature Human Behaviour* 6: 1183.

Barnett, Josephine, Stephanie Aguilar, Mindy Brittner, and Karen Bonuck. 2012. Recruiting and retaining low-income, multi-ethnic women into randomized controlled trials: Successful strategies and staffing. *Contemporary Clinical Trials* 33 (5): 925–932.

Berg, Sara. 2020. Q&A: Why this Black doctor volunteered for coronavirus vaccine trial. *The American Medical Association.* https://www.ama-assn.org/delivering-care/public-health/qa-why-black-doctor-volunteered-coronavirus-vaccine-trial. Accessed June 5, 2021.

Berkowitz, Victoria. 2017. Common courtesy: How the Common Rule strengthens human subject protection. *Houston Law Review* 54: 923–962.

Boden-Albala, Bernadette, Heather Carman, Lauren Southwick, Nina S. Parikh, Eric Roberts, Salina Waddy, and Dorothy Edwards. 2015. Examining barriers and practices to recruitment and retention in stroke clinical trials. *Stroke* 46 (8): 2232–2237.

Brandt, Allan M. 1978. Racism and research: The case of the Tuskegee Syphilis study. *The Hastings Center Report* 8 (6): 21–29.

Branson, Richard D., Kenneth Davis, Jr., and Karyn L. Butler. 2007. African Americans' participation in clinical research: Importance, barriers, and solutions. *The American Journal of Surgery* 193 (1): 32–39.

Eskew, Kevin, Draco Forte, Heidi Haas, Michael India, Erin Atkins Janssen, Scott Lipkin, F. Lisa Murtha, Mary Ann Northrup, Nick Repucci, Rachel Romba, Aysha Somasundaram, and Kayla Tabela. 2013. *The regulation and management of clinical research.* Washington, DC: The Bureau of National Affairs, Inc.

Friedman, David J., and Martin R. Pollak. 2016. Apolipoprotein L1 and kidney disease in African Americans. *Trends in Endocrinology and Metabolism: TEM* 27 (4): 204–215.

Gamble, Justin. 2023. Estate of Henrietta Lacks reaches settlement with biotech company for nonconsensual use of her cells in medical research. *CNN*. https://www.cnn.com/2023/08/01/us/henrietta-lacks-thermo-fisher-scientific-settlement/index.html. Accessed August 5, 2023.

Genovese, G., D.J. Friedman, M.D. Ross, L. Lecordier, P. Uzureau, B.I. Freedman, D.W. Bowden, C.D. Langefeld, T.K. Oleksyk, A.L. Uscinski Knob, A.J. Bernhardy, P.J. Hicks, G.W. Nelson, B. Vanhollebeke, C.A. Winkler, J.B. Kopp, E. Pays, and M.R. Pollak. 2010. Association of trypanolytic ApoL1 variants with kidney disease in African Americans. *Science* 329 (5993): 841–845.

Goodman, Howard. 1998. Studying prison experiments research: For 20 years, a dermatologist used the inmates of a Philadelphia prison as the willing subjects of tests on shampoo, foot powder, deodorant, and later, mind-altering drugs and dioxin. *Knight Ridder/Tribune.* http://articles.baltimoresun.com/1998-07-21/news/1998202099_1_holmesburg-prison-kligman-philadelphia. Accessed August 5, 2023.

Hamel, Lauren, Louis A. Penner, Terrance L. Albrecht, Elisabeth Heath, Clement K. Gwede, and Susan Eggly. 2016. Barriers to clinical trial enrollment in racial and ethnic minority patients with cancer. *Cancer Control* 23 (4): 327–337.

Heller, Jean. 2017. AP was there: Black men untreated in Tuskegee Syphilis study. *APNews.* https://apnews.com/article/race-and-ethnicity-african-americans-medical-research-syphilis-bill-clinton-e9dd07eaa4e74052878a68132cd3803a. Accessed August 5, 2023.

Hornblum, Allen M. 1998. *Acres of skin: Human experiments at Holmsburg prison.* New York: Routledge.

Hudson, Kathy, and Francis S. Collins. 2013. Biospecimen policy: Family matters. *Nature* 500 (7461): 141–142.

Hughes, Travonia B., Vijay R. Varma, Corrinne Pettigrew, and Marilyn S. Albert. 2017. African Americans and clinical research: Evidence concerning barriers and facilitators to participation and recruitment recommendations. *The Gerontologist* 57 (2): 348–358.

Jennings, Madison. 2017. Protected genetics: A case for property and privacy interest in one's own genetic material. *Richmond Journal of Law and Technology* 23: 10–16.

Johns Hopkins Medicine. n.d. The legacy of Henrietta Lacks: Upholding the highest bioethical standards. https://www.hopkinsmedicine.org/henriettalacks/upholding-the-highest-bioethical-standards.html. Accessed August 5, 2023.

Khalil, L., M. Leary, N. Rouphael, I. Ofotokun, P.A. Rebolledo, and Z. Wiley. 2022. Racial and ethnic diversity in SARS-CoV-2 vaccine clinical trials conducted in the United States. *Vaccines (Basel)* 10 (2): 290.

Lewis, Tanya. 2021.The biggest barriers to COVID vaccination for Black and Latinx people. *Scientific American.* https://www.scientificamerican.com/article/the-biggest-barriers-to-covid-vaccination-for-black-and-latinx-people1/. Accessed June 4, 2021.

Limou, Sophie, George W. Wilson, Jeffrey B. Kopp, and Cheryl A. Winkler. 2014. APOL1 kidney risk alleles: Population genetics and disease association. *Advances in Chronic Kidney Disease and Health* 21 (5): 426–433.

Loree, J.M., S. Anand, A. Dasari, J.M. Unger, A. Gothwal, L.M. Ellis, G. Varadhachary, S. Kopetz, M.J. Overman, and K. Raghav. 2019. Disparity of race reporting and representation in clinical trials leading to cancer drug approvals from 2008 to 2018. *JAMA Oncology* 5 (10): e191870.

Luebbert, Rebecca, and Amelia Perez. 2016. Barrier to research participation among African Americans. *Journal of Transcultural Nursing* 27 (5): 456–463.

McKie, Robin. 2010. Henrietta Lacks' cells were priceless, but her family can't afford a hospital. *The Guardian.* https://www.theguardian.com/world/2010/apr/04/henrietta-lacks-cancer-cells. Accessed August 5, 2023.

Mega, Jessica L., Tabassome Simon, Jean-Philippe Collet, Jeffrey L. Anderson, Elliott M. Antman, Kevin Bliden, Christopher P. Cannon, Nicolas Danchin, Betti Giusti, Paul Gurbel, Benjamin D. Horne, Jean-Sebastian Hulot, Adnan Kastrati, Gilles Montalescot, Franz-Josef Neumann, Lei Shen, Dirk Sibbing, P. Gabriel Steg, Dietmar Trenk, Stephen D. Wiviott, and Marc S. Sabatine. 2010. Reduced-function CYP2C19 genotype and risk of adverse clinical outcomes among patients treated with clopidogrel predominantly for PCI: A meta-analysis. *JAMA* 304 (16): 1821–1830.

Mohatt, Nathaniel Vincent, Azure B. Thompson, Nghi D. Thai, and Jacob Kraemer Tebes. 2014. Historical trauma as public narrative: A conceptual review of how history impacts present-day health. *Social Science & Medicine* 106: 128–136.

Oh, Sam S., Joshua Galanter, Neeta Thakur, Maria Pino-Yanes, Nicolas E. Barcelo, Marquitta J. White, Danielle M. de Bruin, Ruth M. Greenblatt, Kirsten Bibbins-Domingo, Alan H. B. Wu, Luisa N. Borrell, Chris Gunter, Neil R. Powe, and Esteban G. Burchard. 2015. Diversity in clinical and biomedical research: A promise yet to be fulfilled. *PLoS Medicine* 12 (12): e1001918.

Parsa, Afshin, W.H. Linda Kao, Dawei Xie, Brad C. Astor, Man Li, Chi-Yuan Hsu, Harold I. Feldman, et al. 2013. APOL1 risk variants, race, and progression of chronic kidney disease. *New England Journal of Medicine* 369: 2183–2196.

Piña, K.R., and W.L. Pines. 2014. *A practical guide to FDA's food and drug law and regulation.* Food and Drug Law Institute, FDLI.

Presidential Commission for the Study of Bioethical Issues. 2011. Ethically impossible: STD research in Guatemala from 1946 to 1948. https://law.stanford.edu/wp-content/uploads/2011/09/EthicallyImpossible_PCSBI_110913.pdf. Accessed August 15, 2023.

Rao, Radhika. 2016. Informed consent, body property, and self-sovereignty. *Journal of Law, Medicine & Ethics* 44: 437–437.

Robbins, William. 1993. Dioxin tests conducted in 60's on 70 Philadelphia inmates, now unknown. *The New York Times*. http://www.nytimes.com/1983/07/17/us/dioxin-tests-conducted-in-60-s-on-70-philadelphia-inmates-now-unknown.html. Accessed August 5, 2023.

Rodriguez, Michael A., and Robert Garcia. 2013. First, do no harm: The U.S. sexually transmitted disease experiments in Guatemala. *American Journal of Public Health* 12 (103): 2122–2126.

Rubin, Susan R. 2014. The clinical trials nurse as subject advocate for minority and culturally diverse research subjects. *Journal of Transcultural Nursing* 25 (4): 383–387.

Sacks, Tina K., Katie Savin, and Quenette L. Walton. 2021. How ancestral trauma informs patients' health decision making. *AMA Journal of Ethics* 23 (2): E183–E188.

Skene, Lea, and Sarah Brumfield. 2023. Henrietta Lacks' family settles lawsuit with a biotech company that used her cells without consent. https://apnews.com/article/henrietta-lacks-hela-cells-thermo-fisher-scientific-bfba4a6c10396efa34c9b79a544f0729. Accessed August 5, 2023.

Skloot, Rebecca. 2010. *The immortal life of Henrietta Lacks*. New York: Random House.

Sotero, Michelle. 2006. A conceptual model of historical trauma: Implications for public health practice and research. *Journal of Health Disparities Research and Practice* 1 (1): 93–108.

Sullivan, Louis. 2002. A conversation with Dr. Louis Sullivan. *Nova Law Review*. https://nsuworks.nova.edu/cgi/viewcontent.cgi?referer=https://www.google.com/&httpsredir=1&article=1333&context=nlr. Accessed August 5, 2023.

The Society for Women's Health Research and the U.S. Food and Drug Administration Office of Women's Health. 2011. Dialogues on diversifying clinical trials: Successful strategies for engaging women and minorities in clinical trials. https://www.fda.gov/files/sciencepercent20&percent20research/published/White-Paper-on-the-Dialogues-on-Diversifying-Clinical-Trials-Conference.pdf. Accessed June 4, 2021.

The White House, Office of the Press Secretary. 1997. Remarks by the president in apology for study done in Tuskegee. https://clintonwhitehouse4.archives.gov/textonly/New/Remarks/Fri/19970516-898.html. Accessed August 5, 2023.

Turner, Tatyana, and Yvonne Wenger. 2020. For the greater good: Black leaders in Baltimore work to overcome resistance to participating in COVID trials, other research. *The Baltimore Sun*. https://www.baltimoresun.com/health/bs-hs-medical-trials-black-participants-20201204-met4kx36srhendn2vznng7eavm-story.html. Accessed June 5, 2021.

Tuskegee University. 2023. About the USPHS study. https://www.tuskegee.edu/about-us/centers-of-excellence/bioethics-center/about-the-usphs-syphilis-study. Accessed August 5, 2023.

U.S. Census Bureau. 2023. Quick facts, United States. https://www.census.gov/quickfacts/fact/table/US/RHI125219. Accessed August 15, 2023.

U.S. Department of Health and Human Services. 2018. 2,3,7,8-Tetrachlorodibenzo-p-dioxin, report on carcinogens. *National Toxicology Program*. https://ntp.niehs.nih.gov/ntp/roc/content/profiles/tetrachlorodibenzodioxin.pdf. Accessed August 5, 2023.

U.S. Department of Health and Human Services, Administration for Children and Families. n.d. Resource guide to trauma-informed human services—What is historical trauma? https://www.acf.hhs.gov/trauma-toolkit/trauma-concept. Accessed May 29, 2023.

U.S. Department of Health and Human Services, Centers for Disease Control and Prevention. 2022a. What is syphilis? CDC basic factsheet. https://www.cdc.gov/std/syphilis/stdfact-syphilis.htm. Accessed August 5, 2023.

U.S. Department of Health and Human Services, Centers for Disease Control and Prevention. 2022b. U.S. Public Health Service syphilis study at Tuskegee. https://www.cdc.gov/tuskegee/timeline.htm. Accessed August 5, 2023.

U.S. Department of Health and Human Services, Centers for Disease Control and Prevention. 2023a. Congenital syphilis—CDC factsheet. https://www.cdc.gov/std/syphilis/stdfact-congenital-syphilis.htm. Accessed August 5, 2023.

U.S. Department of Health and Human Services, Centers for Disease Control and Prevention. 2023b. U.S. Public Health Service syphilis study at Tuskegee. https://www.cdc.gov/tuskegee/index.html. Accessed August 5, 2023.

U.S. Department of Health and Human Services, Centers for Disease Control and Prevention. 2023c. Frequently asked questions. https://www.cdc.gov/tuskegee/faqs.htm. Accessed August 5, 2023.

U.S. Department of Health and Human Services, National Institutes of Health. 2022. NIH clinical research trials and you: The basics. https://www.nih.gov/health-information/nih-clinical-research-trials-you/basics. Accessed August 5, 2023.

U.S. Department of Health and Human Services, National Institute on Minority Health and Health Disparities, National Institutes of Health. 2023. Diversity and inclusion in clinical trials. https://www.nimhd.nih.gov/resources/understanding-health-disparities/diversity-and-inclusion-in-clinical-trials.html. Accessed August 5, 2023.

U.S. Department of Health and Human Services, Office for Human Research Protections. 2023. Revised common rule. https://www.hhs.gov/ohrp/regulations-and-policy/regulations/finalized-revisions-common-rule/index.html. Accessed August 21, 2023.

U.S. Department of Health and Human Services, Office of Minority Health. 2020. Hepatitis and Asian Americans. https://www.minorityhealth.hhs.gov/omh/browse.aspx?lvl=4&lvlid=50. Accessed August 5, 2023.

U.S. Department of Health and Human Services, Office of Minority Health. 2021a. Heart disease and American Indians/Alaska Natives. https://www.minorityhealth.hhs.gov/omh/browse.aspx?lvl=4&lvlid=34. Accessed August 5, 2023.

U.S. Department of Health and Human Services, Office of Minority Health. 2021b. Diabetes and Hispanic Americans. https://www.minorityhealth.hhs.gov/omh/browse.aspx?lvl=4&lvlid=63. Accessed August 5, 2023.

U.S. Department of Health and Human Services, Office of Minority Health. 2021c. Infant mortality and Native Hawaiians/Pacific Islanders. https://www.minorityhealth.hhs.gov/omh/browse.aspx?lvl=4&lvlid=83. Accessed August 5, 2023.

U.S. Department of Health and Human Services, Office of Minority Health. 2023. Stroke and African Americans. https://www.minorityhealth.hhs.gov/omh/browse.aspx?lvl=4&lvlid=28. Accessed August 5, 2023.

U.S. Department of Health, Education, and Welfare, Public Health Service. 1973. Final report of the Tuskegee syphilis study ad hoc advisory panel. https://biotech.law.lsu.edu/cphl/history/reports/tuskegee/completepercent20report.pdf. Accessed June 5, 2021.

U.S. Food and Drug Administration. 2018. What are the different types of clinical research? https://www.fda.gov/ForPatients/ClinicalTrials/Types/default.htm. Accessed June 5, 2021.

U.S. Food and Drug Administration. 2020. Conducting clinical trials. https://www.fda.gov/Drugs/DevelopmentApprovalProcess/ConductingClinicalTrials/default.htm. Accessed June 5, 2021.

U.S. Senate Hearings Before the Subcommittee on Health of the Committee on Labor and Public Welfare Quality of Health Care—Human experimentation. 1973. In *Hearings, Ninety-Third Congress, First Session, on S. 974 ... S. 878 ... S.J. Res. 71 ... 3.*

Vespa, Jonathan, Lauren Medina, and David M. Armstrong. 2020. *Demographic turning points for the United States: Population projections for 2020 to 2060*. U.S. Census Bureau. https://www.census.gov/content/dam/Census/library/publications/2020/demo/p25-1144.pdf. Accessed May 31, 2021.

Vickers, Selwyn M., and Mona N. Fouad. 2014. An overview of EMPaCT and fundamental issues affecting minority participation in cancer clinical trials: Enhancing minority participation in clinical trials (EMPaCT): Laying the groundwork for improving minority clinical trial accrual. *Cancer* 120 (Suppl 7): 1087–1090.

Wendler, Raynard Kington, Jennifer Madans, Gretchen Van Wye, Heidi Christi-Schmidt, Laura A. Pratt, Otis W. Brawley, Cary P. Gross, and Ezekiel Emanuel. 2006. Are racial and ethnic minorities less willing to participate in health research? *PLoS Medicine* 3 (2): e19.

Williams, Erin D. 2005. *CRS report for Congress: Federal protection for human research subjects: An analysis of the common rule and its interactions with FDA regulations and the HIPAA privacy rule*. The Library of Congress. https://fas.org/sgp/crs/misc/RL32909.pdf. Accessed August 5, 2023.

Williams, Harriet A. 2008. *Medical apartheid: The dark history of medical experimentation on black Americans from colonial times to the present*. New York: Random House.

Zimmer, Carl. 2013. A family consents to a medical gift, 62 years later. *The New York Times*. http://www.nytimes.com/2013/08/08/science/after-decades-of-research-henrietta-lacks-family-is-asked-for-consent.html. Accessed August 5, 2023.

Chapter 4
The Impact of Implicit Bias on Data Diversity

Abstract Implicit bias is unconscious stereotypical beliefs or attitudes about a racial or ethnic group and the automatic preference for a particular group. Health care provider implicit bias may contribute to health disparities because it influences clinical, diagnostic and treatment decisions, patient-provider communication, patient adherence to treatment recommendations, and treatment outcomes. Moreover, implicit bias may lead to different clinical decisions for patients with the same clinical symptoms, thereby affecting disease outcomes. When a patient is not provided a specific treatment, is excluded from treatment protocol, or not referred to a clinical trial because of these biases, it may have data implications. This chapter discusses implicit bias and how it may limit clinical trial participation and impact data quality. Section 4.1 defines implicit bias. Section 4.2 explores research on implicit bias. Section 4.3 discusses data bias and clinical trials. Section 4.4 summarizes key points in this chapter.

Keywords Implicit bias · Explicit bias · Clinical trials · Clinical decision-making · Pain management · Cardiovascular disease

4.1 What Is Implicit Bias?

Bias impacts our interactions, perceptions, and how we think and process information. Data are susceptible to these perceptions as well as the knowledge, experiences, and biases of the person who labels and collects them. Similarly, a physician's perceptions and bias can impact their interaction with the patient (Hamel et al. 2016; Marshall and Palokoff 2023). There are many types of bias, including historical, racial, cultural, sexual, gender, disability, ageism, socioeconomic, and implicit. There is also explicit bias—or overt bigotry—that is conscious and controllable (Maina et al. 2017). One way that bias is infused in algorithms is when those biases are embedded in the datasets used to train the algorithm (Benjamin 2019). This can lead to the algorithm producing a prejudiced result (Benjamin 2019). Implicit bias is unconscious stereotypical beliefs or attitudes about a racial or ethnic minority group

N. H. Williams, *Artificial Intelligence and Healthcare*, The International Library of Bioethics 107, https://doi.org/10.1007/978-3-031-48262-5_4

and the automatic preference for a particular group (Hagiwara et al. 2020; Haider et al. 2015). It is learned through individual experiences and the perceptions and interactions with one own's social group (Haider et al. 2015). In the clinical setting, implicit bias can manifest itself as attitudes and stereotypes toward racial and ethnic minority patients (Haider et al. 2015).

In 2003, the Institute of Medicine (IOM)[1] published the landmark report, *Unequal Treatment: Confronting Racial and Ethnic Disparities in Health Care.* This report examined the racial and ethnic differences in health care, their potential sources, and recommendations to eliminate these disparities (Institute of Medicine (US) Committee on Understanding and Eliminating Racial and Ethnic Disparities in Health Care 2003). The IOM report found that racial and ethnic disparities in health care were endemic throughout health care services to treat various illnesses, regardless of socioeconomic and access issues. Some sources of these disparities included systemic barriers, health care providers, patients, and bias (Institute of Medicine (US) Committee on Understanding and Eliminating Racial and Ethnic Disparities in Health Care 2003). Additionally, the report found that physician implicit bias may contribute to health disparities because it influences clinical and diagnostic decisions and patient treatment recommendations (Institute of Medicine (US) Committee on Understanding and Eliminating Racial and Ethnic Disparities in Health Care 2003).

The National Healthcare Quality and Disparities Report (NHQDR) is an annual report that assesses the strengths, weaknesses, disparities, access, and quality of the U.S. health care system (U.S. Department of Health and Human Services. Agency for Healthcare Research and Quality 2020) The 2019 report found that "Blacks and American Indians and Alaska Natives received worse care than Whites for about 40% of quality measures; Hispanics received worse care than non-Hispanic Whites for about 35% of quality measures; and Asians and Native Hawaiians/Pacific Islanders received worse care than Whites for about 30% of quality measures, but Asians also received better care for about 30% of quality measures." (U.S. Department of Health and Human Services. Agency for Healthcare Research and Quality 2020, p. D5). The report found that disparities in health care may "occur for a variety of reasons including differences in access to care, social determinants, provider biases, poor provider-patient communication, and poor health literacy." (U.S. Department of Health and Human Services. Agency for Healthcare Research and Quality 2020, p. D1).

Because implicit bias is unconscious and subtle, it is also more insidious. Most people, including health care providers, are not overtly racist, but they may harbor unconscious biases (Marshall and Palokoff 2023). Their views are shaped by many factors, including their experiences, culture, family, religion, and societal messages and attitudes. However, these perceptions may inadvertently manifest themselves in racist beliefs or behaviors. Many people, including health care providers, may not be

[1] The National Academy of Medicine (NAM) was founded as the Institute of Medicine (IOM) in 1970. IOM's name was changed in 2015 to NAM. NAM, the National Academy of Sciences, and the National Academy of Engineering, comprise the National Academies in the United States. The National Academies are nonprofit, private organizations that provide independent and expert scientific advice to inform policy.

aware that they hold these attitudes, perceptions, or stereotypes (Institute of Medicine (US) Committee on Understanding and Eliminating Racial and Ethnic Disparities in Health Care. 2003).

> These biases have their origins in normal and pervasive processes associated with social categorization and thus can operate without conscious awareness or control. Whether consciously endorsed or not, stereotypes are heuristics that typically efficiently guide the perception, interpretation, storage, and retrieval of information, particularly under conditions of high cognitive demand....Similarly, when individuals do not have the time, capacity, opportunity, or motivation to assess situations fully and deliberately, implicit attitudes automatically shape people's responses to objects, individuals, and groups. These conditions of time pressure, high cognitive demand, and stress are common to many health care settings, making these settings "ripe" to activate stereotypes (Institute of Medicine (US) Committee on Understanding and Eliminating Racial and Ethnic Disparities in Health Care. 2003, p. 173).

In a systematic literature review, researchers found that many health care providers, regardless of specialty, training, and experience, harbored negative attitudes toward people of color (i.e., Blacks, Hispanics, Latinos, and individuals with dark skin) and positive attitudes toward Whites (Hagiwara et al. 2020; Hall et al. 2015; Institute of Medicine (US) Committee on Understanding and Eliminating Racial and Ethnic Disparities in Health Care 2003). This implicit bias may lead to different clinical decisions for patients with the same clinical symptoms (Shirey and Morris 2019). Implicit bias unlocks the chance that "medical decisions and the course of treatment will reflect subjective variability and preferences of the physician. Under conditions of time pressure, problem complexity, and high cognitive demand, physicians' attitudes may therefore shape their interpretation of this information and their expectations for treatment, such as the likelihood of patient compliance." (Institute of Medicine (US) Committee on Understanding and Eliminating Racial and Ethnic Disparities in Health Care. 2003, p. 161).

Health care provider implicit bias may manifest itself in verbal and nonverbal cues such as limited time spent with the patient, eye contact, body language, physical contact, and the tone and speed of speech (Hagiwara et al. 2020; Institute of Medicine (US) Committee on Understanding and Eliminating Racial and Ethnic Disparities in Health Care 2003). Additionally, implicit bias may negatively impact communication between the health care provider and patient. Patient-centered communication is correlated with increased patient trust, treatment adherence, and medical care continuity (Cooper et al. 2012; Thomas and Booth-McCoy 2020). It is "eliciting, understanding, and validating the patient's perspective (e.g., concerns, feelings, expectations); understanding the patient within his or her own psychological and social context; reaching a shared understanding of the patient's problem and its treatment; and helping a patient share power by offering him or her meaningful involvement in choices relating to his or her health." (Epstein and Street 2007, p. 2). Research suggests that physician implicit bias may impact their communication with Black patients in the clinical setting (Blair et al. 2013).

In short, health care providers may not realize that they have implicit bias. Their unconscious stereotypical beliefs or attitudes about a racial or ethnic minority group may impact treatment decisions and affect patient-provider communication. It may also affect the health care provider's perception of whether a patient will adhere to treatment recommendations, possibly impacting treatment outcomes. This also impacts data because health care data come from many sources including medical records, clinical trials, and insurance claims, to name a few. If a health care provider's implicit bias impedes communication with the patient about health concerns, the valuable information that could have been learned will not be captured in the medical record. If a health care provider's implicit bias prevents recommending a patient for certain treatment or a clinical trial because they believe the patient would not be compliant, the potential for more robust clinical trial results is lost because the patient was not referred. Thus, implicit bias not only impacts how data are coded but also what data are collected and included.

4.2 Implicit Bias Research

There are various methods to measure implicit bias including the Implicit Association Test (IAT), the Implicit Rational Assessment Procedure (IRAP), and scientific research. IAT measures the strength of unconscious automatic associations between concepts or objects (e.g., Black people, young people, older adults) and evaluations (e.g., good or bad) or stereotypes (e.g., intelligent, reckless, slow) (Greenwald et al. 1998; Project Implicit 2021). The respondent classifies words or pictures into a group representing concepts or objects and evaluations or stereotypes (Blair et al. 2013). The respondent's classification speed determines the strength of the association – the faster the speed, the stronger the association (Blair et al. 2013). The IRAP is a computer-based tool that also measures the strength of association between targeted stimuli and the interrelatedness between the stimuli (Sereno et al. 2021).

Implicit bias has also been explored in numerous research studies. Schulman et al. (1999) examined racial and gender differences in the treatment of cardiovascular disease, physician decision-making, and differences in treatment recommendations. The researchers developed a 10-min computerized multimedia survey to collect physician responses to a videotaped interview of a patient with chest pains in order to evaluate physician pain management recommendations, physician opinion of the patients' characteristics, and physician demographic information (Schulman et al. 1999). The researchers developed 144 case studies based upon all possible combinations of race (Black or White), age (55 or 70), sex, exercise stress test results, chest pain type, coronary risk (low or high), and electrocardiogram results (Schulman et al. 1999). Eight actors representing all possible combinations of race, age, and sex were employed to portray patients with chest pain (Schulman et al. 1999). Of the three scripts developed, two reflected the three different types of chest pain—definite angina, possible angina, or nonanginal pain (Schulman et al. 1999). The actors recited the scripts verbatim and used identical hand motions for the interviews. Additionally, the hospital gowns and filmed camera angles remained consistent for each interview (Schulman et al. 1999). The actors represented people with identical insurance and occupations based upon the age. The researchers' goal was to present patients with identical histories, control for personality characteristics, and remove socioeconomic and insurance status as factors (Schulman et al. 1999). As part of the study design and to pretest accuracy, four cardiologists reviewed the videos and classified the type of pain described. Their classifications agreed more than 75% of the time (Schulman et al. 1999).

The study involved 720 full-time clinical practice physicians who attended either the 1996 annual meeting of the American Academy of Family Practice or the 1997 annual American College of Physicians meeting (Schulman et al. 1999). Each physician received background information on the patient (e.g., occupation, type of insurance), viewed the videotaped interview, and then made a treatment recommendation. The researchers discovered that the two factors that independently influenced the physicians' treatment recommendations were the patient's race and gender, regardless of the clinical manifestations of chest pain (Schulman et al. 1999). The researchers suggested that bias may be a factor in the physicians' decision-making but could not determine if the bias was overt or subconscious (Schulman et al. 1999).

In another study, van Ryn and Burke (2000) analyzed approximately 600 surveys of physician–patient encounters post-angiogram treatment. They found that the physicians perceived Black coronary artery disease (CAD) patients to be at risk for substance abuse, noncompliant with medical advice, and have limited social support (van Ryn and Burke 2000). They also perceived the patients to be less educated and intelligent than their White counterparts, despite controlling for age, sex, gender, income, and education (van Ryn and Burke 2000). Furthermore, the physicians felt less affiliation with their Black patients (van Ryn and Burke 2000). The researchers also discovered that low socioeconomic (SES) patients were perceived as less likely to comply with treatment, less likely to desire to be physically active, and less likely to have career demands, family responsibilities, and social supports (van Ryn and Burke 2000). Low SES patients also received negative ratings for intelligence, rationality, and self-control regardless of age, sex, and race (van Ryn and Burke 2000). Consequently, physicians viewed Blacks and low SES populations more negatively than Whites and those in higher socioeconomic levels (van Ryn and Burke 2000).

Breathett et al. (2019) found that race modestly influenced heart transplant decisions. The study utilized clinical vignettes and interviews. Study participants were recruited from a national heart failure organization comprised of postdoctoral trainees, nurses, pharmacists, physicians, and nurse practitioners trained to care for patients with advanced heart failure (Breathett et al. 2019). The clinical vignettes were identical except for race, describing a patient with end-stage heart failure, lack of social support, poor treatment adherence, financial instability, and medical comorbidities such as history of drug abuse, obesity, diabetes, kidney disease, and peripheral vascular disease (Breathett et al. 2019). As the participants reviewed the clinical vignette sections, they were interviewed on patient eligibility for advanced therapies, the final recommendation for the type of advanced therapy, and trustworthiness of the patient (Breathett et al. 2019). After reviewing the vignettes, the participants rated how suitable the patient was for a heart transplant or ventricular assist devices (Breathett et al. 2019). The researchers found that race modestly influenced the decision process for advanced treatment—White patients were recommended to receive heart transplants and Black patients ventricular assisted devices (Breathett et al. 2019). Also, racial bias may be a factor during the interviews (Breathett et al. 2019).

The IOM stated in its 2011 report, *Relieving Pain in America: A Blueprint for Transforming Prevention, Care, Education, and Research,* that stereotyping and bias contributed to significant barriers in pain care and management (Institute of Medicine 2011). In a meta-analysis and systematic review of 20 years of research on racial and ethnic disparities in analgesic pain treatment in the United States, Meghani et al. (2012) found that the risk for undertreatment for minorities was more evident because they were more likely to receive non-opioid analgesics, when compared to Whites. Specifically, Blacks and Hispanics were less likely to receive opioid prescriptions when the source of pain was not easily verifiable (Meghani et al. 2012). Additionally, Blacks were less likely to receive a prescription for opioids and non-opioid analgesics regardless of whether the pain was traumatic (e.g., postoperative, bone fracture) or non-traumatic (e.g., arthritis, migraine, back pain, abdominal pain) (Meghani et al. 2012). In another study, Tamayo-Sarver et al. (2003) analyzed national emergency room data to compare prescriptions of analgesics and opioids by race and ethnicity. They found that Blacks and Latinos were less likely to receive opioids than Whites. Specifically, Blacks were less like to receive opioids for migraine and back pain when compared to Whites. Their findings were consistent with their hypothesis that opioid prescribing requires more physician trust in the patient (Tamayo-Sarver et al. 2003). Likewise, Sabon and Greenwald (2012) found that Black pediatric patients were less likely to receive narcotic pain medication than Whites due to pediatrician implicit bias.

In another study, Hoffman et al. (2016) examined racial bias based upon beliefs about the biological differences between Blacks and Whites. In the two-study design, the researchers examined whether people without medical training and those with some medical training (i.e., medical students and residents) believed that Blacks experienced less pain than Whites (Hoffman et al. 2016). Furthermore, they studied if those with medical training prescribed less pain medication to Blacks than Whites (Hoffman et al. 2016). In study one, White adults without medical training believed that Blacks had a higher pain tolerance than Whites. They falsely assumed that Blacks were physiologically stronger than Whites (Hoffman et al. 2016). In study two, half of the medical students and residents believed the fallacy about biological differences between Blacks and Whites related to pain and that Blacks suffered less pain than Whites (Hoffman et al. 2016). Consequently, this false belief led the medical students and residents to make inaccurate treatment recommendations for Black patients (Hoffman et al. 2016).

Health care provider negative attitudes may also impact who is included in clinical research. For example, a health provider may believe that non-White patients may be poor candidates for clinical trials because they are less likely to adhere to treatment recommendations (Hamel et al. 2016). As a result, racial and ethnic minority groups may be excluded from clinical trial participation. Likewise, if a health care provider unconsciously limits his time with the patient, believes that the patient is non-compliant, or does not engage in patient-centered treatment and communication, he may miss information such as body cues and patient words that may be helpful in diagnosis and treatment. Additionally, a patient who feels that the physician is biased may hold back relevant information that can be important in determining treatment. The implicit or explicit bias has data implications. If a patient is not provided a specific treatment, is excluded from treatment protocol, or is not referred to a clinical trial because of these biases, it can result in missing clinical and research data because the patient is excluded. The algorithms trained with these data can produce a racial and ethnic algorithmic bias due to the lack of data diversity in the sample and the implicit bias buried in the data (Char et al. 2018). The algorithm's predictive capability is compromised if there is little or no data on the target population in the training data. Similarly, the potential for bias occurs in clinical research and trial data because racial and ethnic minority groups are underrepresented in the clinical trials. Therefore, their inclusion in the data is limited. Such data are necessary to train algorithms. Some may argue that statistical techniques such as oversampling or an iterative approach to algorithm construction may correct for such bias (Peek et al. 2014). However, that does not solve the issue that bias still exists (Campolo et al. 2017).

4.3 Why Diversity in Clinical Trials Is Important

Historically, clinical trial data were skewed towards White men, not women or racial and ethnic minority groups (Campolo et al. 2017). Regardless of the reason for this exclusion, be it overt racism, sexism, or the perception that women needed to be protected from research, data training datasets in health care depend upon the use of various data sources, including clinical trial data (Campolo et al. 2017). To identify sex/gender and racial and ethnic differences and determine treatment effectiveness and efficacy, the inclusion of women and racial and ethnic minority groups is crucial. Unfortunately, as discussed in the previous chapter, many racial and ethnic minority groups are hesitant to participate in clinical trials due to mistrust as a result of historical clinical research abuses and malfeasance (Institute of Medicine (US) Committee on Understanding and Eliminating Racial and Ethnic Disparities in Health Care 2003; Scharff et al. 2010). Moreover, bias, both explicit and implicit, may exacerbate mistrust of the health care system and clinical research, limiting the participation of racial and ethnic minority groups in clinical trials, leading them to be excluded in the data collection (Institute of Medicine (US) Committee on Understanding and Eliminating Racial and Ethnic Disparities in Health Care 2003; Scharff et al. 2010).

As examined in Chap. 3, diversity in clinical trial participation is essential for the validity, generalizability, safety, and efficacy of clinical trial results (Warren et al. 2020). Bhatnagar et al. (2017) found that the median percentage of Blacks in a multiple myeloma[2] clinical trial was only 4.5%, despite this population representing 20% of multiple myeloma cases (Bhatnagar et al. 2017). The researchers surmised that increased participation of Blacks in clinical trials would improve access to new treatment therapies, the trials would be representative of the U.S. population, and the data produced would provide insights on the disease impacts on Blacks, possibly identifying molecular and clinical characteristics that can be targeted by particular drug therapies (Bhatnagar et al. 2017). ProPublica, an investigative non-profit newsroom, found that Blacks were under-represented in new drug clinical trials for multiple myeloma, which affects Blacks two to three times higher than Whites. Of the 722 clinical trial participants, only 1.8% were Black (Morra 2018). ProPublica also discovered that Blacks comprised fewer than 5% of clinical trial participants in 24 of 31 cancer drugs approved by the U.S. Food and Drug Administration (FDA) since 2015 (Morra 2018). Other racial and ethnic groups were also not represented. For example, Asians, which made up approximately 6% of the U.S. population, accounted for 1.7% of the clinical trial participants, of which 70% of the studies were conducted in the United States (Morra 2018). Additionally, Native Americans or Alaska Natives were not reported in approximately two-thirds of the clinical trials despite being 2% of the U.S. population (Morra 2018).

In 1998, FDA recognizing the lack of diversity in clinical trials based on age groups, gender, and race, issued the Final Rule on Investigational New Drug Applications and New Drug Applications, otherwise known as the Demographic Rule (Auderset 2018). It required new drug applications to include summaries of effectiveness and safety data for racial subgroups. In addition, it required sponsors to include information on demographic subgroup clinical trial participation according to age, gender, and race in annual reports (U.S. Food and Drug Administration 1998). The FDA amended its regulations because different subgroups may react differently to clinical interventions, and there may be differences in effectiveness and adverse reactions (U.S. Food and Drug Administration 1998).

> This final rule reflects the growing recognition within the agency and the health community that: (1) Different subgroups of the population may respond differently to a specific drug product and (2) although the effort should be made to look for differences in effectiveness and adverse reactions among such subgroups that effort is not being made consistently.
>
> Since the early 1980's, FDA has been concerned about possible differences in response to drugs among subsets of the overall population, such as age, gender, or racial subsets. The agency has addressed in various ways the question of how to obtain information that would permit individualization of therapy. Evaluation of potential differences among demographic subsets requires that individuals from these subsets be included in studies and that analyses to seek differences in response be carried out. During the past decade, FDA has encouraged demographic subgroup analyses in various guidance documents and other regulatory actions. FDA also has examined the extent of participation of patient subgroups in drug development programs (U.S. Food and Drug Administration 1998).

[2] Multiple myeloma is a blood cancer.

In July 2012, the Food and Drug Administration Safety and Innovation Act of 2012 (FDASIA) was signed into law.[3] The law amended the Federal Food, Drug, and Cosmetic Act to reauthorize user fee programs for prescription drugs and medical devices; establish user fee programs for generic human drugs and biosimilars; and made other changes to improve the regulatory process for medical devices.[4] The law also required recommendations to improve the completeness and quality of analysis on demographic subgroups data.[5] Section 907, titled *Reporting of Inclusion of Demographic Subgroups in Clinical Trials and Data Analysis in Applications for Drugs, Biologics, and Devices*, required FDA to publish a report addressing this issue to ensure that "clinical trial participation and the inclusion of safety and effectiveness data by demographic subgroups including sex, age, race, and ethnicity, is included in applications submitted to the Food and Drug Administration, and shall provide such publication to Congress."[6] One year after the publication of the report, FDA was required to publish an action plan with recommendations to improve the completeness and quality of data on demographic subgroups, include and make available such data on labeling, and improve the public availability of such data.[7] The FDASIA 907 report, published in August 2013, found that.

> The overall findings showed that Whites represented a high percentage of trial participants, which may in part reflect lower percentages of non-White racial demographic subgroups in the U.S. population (see Appendix 3). For some of the indications, race composition in the trials was consistent with the disease prevalence (e.g., melanoma and head lice are more prevalent in Whites). However, for other indications, race composition was not consistent with disease prevalence in the U.S. population, and African American representation was low relative to the African American population with the disease. For example, for type 2 diabetes mellitus (T2DM), African American representation in clinical studies was less than 5%, even though African Americans make up approximately 13% of the U.S. population and have a higher prevalence of T2DM (U.S. Food and Drug Administration 2013, p. 18).

As required by FDASIA, FDA released its Action Plan for FDASIA Section 907 in August 2014 (U.S. Food and Drug Administration 2014). In the Action Plan, FDA's three priorities were: "to improve the completeness and quality of demographic subgroup data; identify barriers to subgroup enrollment in clinical trials and employ strategies to encourage greater participation; and make demographic subset data more available and transparent." (U.S. Food and Drug Administration 2014, p. 2). The FDA acknowledged that the Action Plan was the first step in a process to include diverse populations in clinical research stating, "Greater representation of

[3] U.S. Food and Drug Administration Safety and Innovation Act of 2012, Pub. L. 112-144, § 126 Stat. 993.

[4] U.S. Food and Drug Administration Safety and Innovation Act of 2012, Pub. L. 112–144, § 126 Stat. 993.

[5] U.S. Food and Drug Administration Safety and Innovation Act of 2012, Pub. L. 112–144, § 126 Stat. 993, 1094.

[6] U.S. Food and Drug Administration Safety and Innovation Act of 2012, Pub. L. 112–144, § 126 Stat. 993, 1092–1093.

[7] U.S. Food and Drug Administration Safety and Innovation Act of 2012, Pub. L. 112–144, § 126 Stat. 993.

diverse populations in applications for FDA-regulated medical products is beneficial. By improving data quality, encouraging greater participation in clinical trials, and making demographic subgroup data more available and transparent, we can help to ensure that researchers, health professionals, and consumers will have easy access to meaningful clinical information about medical products that will help them make informed decisions." (U.S. Food and Drug Administration 2014, p. 17). However, FDA did not recommend the mandatory inclusion of a certain number or percentage of demographic subgroups in their clinical trials.

In October 2016, FDA released its guidance titled *Collection of Race and Ethnicity Data in Clinical Trials* (U.S. Food and Drug Administration 2016). The guidance stated FDA's expectation that sponsors will enroll clinical trial participants "who reflect the demographics for clinically relevant populations regarding age, gender, race, and ethnicity" (U.S. Food and Drug Administration 2016, p. 3). However, it did not mandate a level of participation. In September 2017, FDA released its guidance titled *Evaluation and Reporting of Age-, Race, and Ethnicity Specific Data in Medical Device Clinical Studies* (U.S. Food and Drug Administration 2017). The guidance recommended that "to achieve an unbiased estimate of treatment effect in the general population, sponsors should develop a strategy to enroll diverse populations including representative proportions of relevant age, racial, and ethnic subgroups, which are consistent with the intended use population of the device." (U.S. Food and Drug Administration 2017, p. 5). Furthermore, if there is insufficient demographic subgroup data to assess clinically meaningful outcomes, FDA may determine that additional clinical data from the demographic subgroups "may be needed pre- or post-market to address potential age-, race-, or ethnicity-specific questions related to safety or effectiveness in any or all of those subgroups." (U.S. Food and Drug Administration 2017, p. 26).

Even though diversity in clinical trials is an FDA priority, the guidance does not have the operation of law (U.S. Food and Drug Administration 2017). FDA recommendations describe the agency's rationale on a topic but are nonbinding unless there are specific regulatory or statutory requirements (Auderset 2018). FDA may deny the pre- or post-marketing of devices if the demographic subgroup data are insufficient, but it is not a statutory or regulatory requirement (U.S. Food and Drug Administration 2017). For Class III medical devices, FDA requires the submission and approval of a pre-market approval (PMA) application to ensure safety and effectiveness before a device can be marketed (U.S. Food and Drug Administration 2019). Class III devices must receive pre-market approval to ensure safety and efficacy because they are life-sustaining, life-supporting, or new devices that are not equivalent to anything on the market. However, in a study examining the enrollment reporting of race, ethnicity, gender, and age, researchers found that for 2015 PMA devices, race and ethnicity were only reported for half of the studies (Dhruva et al. 2017). Moreover, fewer than 20% of the PMAs analyzed provided results for age, race and/or ethnicity, and/or sex (Dhruva et al. 2017). Similarly, in a separate research study that examined FDA-approved novel therapeutics between 2011 and 2013, researchers found that the participation of Blacks and Hispanics in pivotal trials was low considering their representation in the general population (Downing et al. 2016). Additionally, the participation of Blacks was very low considering the rates of disease burden in minority populations from diseases like cancer, heart disease, and diabetes (Downing et al. 2016). Consequently, racial disparities in clinical trials were still prevailing (Downing et al. 2016).

In 2020, the FDA published its final guidance titled *Enhancing the Diversity of Clinical Trial Populations—Eligibility, Criteria, Enrollment Practices, and Trial Designs.* It encouraged clinical trial sponsors to enroll participants "who reflect the characteristics of clinically relevant populations with regard to age, sex, race, and ethnicity." (U.S. Food and Drug Administration 2020, p. 5) Regarding racial and ethnic minorities, the guidance states:

> Differences in response to medical products (e.g., pharmacokinetics, efficacy, or safety) have been observed in racially and ethnically distinct subgroups of the U.S. population. These differences may be attributable to intrinsic factors (e.g., genetics, metabolism, elimination), extrinsic factors (e.g., diet, environmental exposure, sociocultural issues), or interactions between these factors. Analyzing data on race and ethnicity may assist in identifying population-specific signals. Therefore, FDA recommends that for drugs and biologics, sponsors include a plan for inclusion of clinically relevant populations (U.S. Food and Drug Administration 2020, pp. 6–7).

This guidance also encourages geographic diversity in clinical trials, as well as diversity in selecting health care professionals and study coordinators. Specifically, the guidance states that "clinical trial sites include geographic locations with a higher concentration of racial and ethnic minority patients and indigenous populations, as well as locations within the neighborhoods where these populations receive their health care, because restricting clinical trial sites to selected geographic locations may limit the ability to enroll a diverse trial population. Consider diversity when selecting health care providers and study coordinators to assist with clinical trial recruitment, because participants may prefer a health care provider of their same cultural background." (U.S. Food and Drug Administration 2020, p. 11).

In 2022, FDA issued draft guidance titled *Diversity Plans to Improve Enrollment of Participants from Underrepresented Racial and Ethnic Populations in Clinical Trials;Guidance for Industry.* It expands the 2016 guidance, recommending that sponsors develop a Race and Ethnicity Diversity Plan. Once again, recognizing the importance of diversity in clinical research, health disparities, and health care access, the FDA guidance "outlines how to collect and present race and ethnicity data in submissions to the FDA and recommends that sponsors develop and submit a plan to address inclusion of clinically relevant populations, for discussion to the Agency. …. FDA recommends that a Plan to enroll representative numbers of participants from historically underrepresented racial and ethnic populations be submitted to the investigational new drug (IND) application, for a drug, including biological products regulated as drugs, or the investigational device exemption (IDE) application, for a device" (U.S. Food and Drug Administration 2022, p. 2).

Critics argue that "legislating demographics" overburdens the system because it is challenging to recruit clinical trial participants, regardless of race and ethnicity

(Auderset 2018). In addition, clinical studies vary greatly, and a blanket percentage or mandatory number is unrealistic (Auderset 2018). On the contrary, mandatory minimums for clinical trial participation will ensure safety and efficacy for the diverse U.S. population because the data would be inclusive and generalizable (Boden-Albala et al. 2015). Equally important, it would enhance medical artificial intelligence's predictive value because the data would be inclusive of diverse groups and generalizable (Branson et al. 2007; Zhang et al. 2017). Lastly, as stated previously, some research has shown that racial and ethnic minority groups are just as willing to participate in clinical trials as Whites, but they are not asked to do so (Wendler et al. 2006).

4.4 Summary

Bias, whether explicit or implicit, affects treatment outcomes, treatment decisions, patient-physician interactions, and clinical decisions (Burgess et al. 2017; Metzl et al. 2017). The implicit biases that are embedded in the health care system perpetuate the racial disparities and ethnic disparities in health care and health outcomes (Metzl et al. 2017). If a patient is not provided a specific treatment, is excluded from treatment protocol, or is not referred to a clinical trial because of these biases, it can result in missing clinical and research data because the patient is excluded. Data must be trustworthy, accurate, and timely. They also must be inclusive and without bias (Zhang et al. 2017). Data bias occurs when data from certain populations are missing, and the incomplete data are encoded into training datasets. It is imperative to capture and incorporate data from racial and ethnic minority groups. If data are not representative and diverse, then the output of the algorithmic model may be biased, resulting in flawed predictive capability and ineffective algorithmic models.

References

Auderset, Megan. 2018. FDA guidance recommends diversity in clinical trials, but can't require it. *Journal for Clinical Studies.* 12: 12–15.

Benjamin, Ruha. 2019. Assessing risk, automating racism. *Science* 366 (6464): 421–422.

Bhatnagar, Vishal, Nicole Gormley, Dickran Kazandjian, Kirsten Goldberg, Amy E. McKee, Gideon Blumenthal, Ann T. Farrell, and Richard Pazdur. 2017. FDA analysis of racial demographics in multiple myeloma trials. *Blood* 130 (Suppl1): 4352.

Blair, I.V., John F. Steiner, Diane L. Fairclough, Rebecca Hanratty, David W. Price, Holen K. Hirsh, Leslie A. Wright, Michael Bronsert, Elhum Karimkhani, David J. Magid, and Edward P. Havranek. 2013. Clinicians' implicit ethnic/racial bias and perceptions of care among Black and Latino patients. *The Annals of Family Medicine* 11 (1): 43–52.

Boden-Albala, Bernadette, Heather Carman, Lauren Southwick, Nina S. Parikh, Eric Roberts, Salina Waddy, and Dorothy Edwards. 2015. Examining barriers and practices to recruitment and retention in stroke clinical trials. *Stroke* 46 (8): 2232–2237.

Branson, Richard D., Kenneth Davis, and Karyn L. Butler. 2007. African Americans' participation in clinical research: Importance, barriers, and solutions. *The American Journal of Surgery* 193 (1): 32–39.

Breathett, Khadijah, Erika Yee, Natalie Pool, Megan Hebdon, Janice D. Crist, Shannon Knapp, Ashley Larsen, Sade Solola, Luis Luy, Katherine Herrera-Theut, Leanne Zabala, Jeff Stone, Marylyn M. McEwen, Elizabeth Calhoun, and Nancy K. Sweitzer. 2019. Does race influence decision making for advanced heart failure therapies? *Journal of the American Heart Association* 8 (22): e013592.

Burgess, D.J., M.C. Beach, and S. Saha. 2017. Mindfulness practice: A promising approach to reducing the effects of clinician implicit bias on patients. *Patient Education and Counseling* 100 (2): 372–376.

Campolo, Alex, Madelyn Sanfillippo, Meredith Whittaker, and Kate Crawford. 2017. AI now 2017 report. *AI Now*. https://ainowinstitute.org/publication/ai-now-2017-report-2. Accessed 6 June 2021.

Char, D.S., N.H. Shah, and D. Magnus. 2018. Implementing machine learning in health care: Addressing ethical challenges. *The New England Journal of Medicine* 378 (11): 981–983.

Cooper, L.A., Debra L. Roter, Kathryn A. Carson, Mary Catherine Beach, Janice A. Sabin, G. Greenwald. Anthony, and Thomas S. Inui. 2012. The associations of clinicians' implicit attitudes about race with medical visit communication and patient ratings of interpersonal care. *American Journal of Public Health* 102 (5): 979–987.

Dhruva, Sanket S., Carolyn M. Mazure, Joseph S. Ross, and Rita F. Redberg. 2017. Inclusion of demographic-specific information in studies supporting US food and drug administration approval of high-risk medical devices. *JAMA Internal Medicine*. 177 (9): 1–2.

Downing, N.S., N.D. Shah, J.H. Neiman, J.A. Aminawung, H.M. Krumholz, and J.S. Ross. 2016. Participation of the elderly, women, and minorities in pivotal trials supporting 2011–2013 US food and drug administration approvals. *Trials* 17: 199.

Epstein, R.M., and Richard L. Street. 2007. Patient-centered communication in cancer care: Promoting healing and reducing suffering. In *National Cancer Institute/National Institutes of Health Publication*, NIH Publication No. 07-6225 Bethesda, MD. https://cancercontrol.cancer.gov/sites/default/files/2020-06/pcc_monograph.pdf. Accessed 15 Feb 2021.

Greenwald, A.G., Debbie E. McGhee, and Jordan L.K.. Schwartz. 1998. Measuring individual differences in implicit cognition: The implicit association test. *Journal of Personality and Social Psychology* 74 (6): 1464–1480.

Hagiwara, N., Frederick W. Kron, Mark W. Scerbo, and Ginger S. Watson. 2020. A call for grounding implicit bias training in clinical and translational frameworks. *Lancet* 395 (10234): 1457–1460.

Haider, A.H., E.B. Schneider, N. Sriram, V.K. Scott, S.M. Swoboda, C.K. Zogg, N. Dhiman, E.R. Haut, D.T. Efron, P.J. Pronovost, J.A. Freischlag, P.A. Lipsett, E.E. Cornwell, E.J. MacKenzie, and L.A. Cooper. 2015. Unconscious race and class biases among registered nurses: Vignette-based study using implicit association testing. *Journal of the American College of Surgeons* 220 (6): 1077-1086.e3.

Hall, W.J., Mimi V. Chapman, Kent M. Lee, Yesenia M. Merino, Tainayah W. Thomas, B. Keith Payne, Eugenia Eng, Steven H. Day, and Tamera Coyne-Beasley. 2015. Implicit racial/ethnic bias among health care professionals and its influence on health care outcomes: A systematic review. *American Journal of Public Health* 105 (12): e60–e76.

Hamel, Lauren M., Louis A. Penner, Terrance L. Albrecht, Elisabeth Heath, Clement K. Gwede, and Susan Eggly. 2016. Barriers to clinical trial enrollment in racial and ethnic minority patients with cancer. *Cancer Control* 23 (4): 327–337.

Hoffman, K.M., Sophie Trawalter, Jordan R. Axt, and M. Norman Oliver. 2016. Racial bias in Pain assessment and treatment recommendations, and false beliefs about biological differences between blacks and whites. *Proceedings of the National Academy of Sciences* 113 (16): 4296–4301.

Institute of Medicine (US) Committee on Understanding and Eliminating Racial and Ethnic Disparities in Health Care. 2003. *Unequal treatment: confronting racial and ethnic disparities in health care*, eds. B.D. Smedley, A.Y. Stith, A.R. Nelson. Washington DC: National Academies Press.

Institute of Medicine. 2011. *Relieving pain in America: A blueprint for transforming prevention, care, education, and research.* Washington, DC: National Academies Press.

Maina, Ivy W., Tanisha D. Belton, Sara Ginzberg, Ajit Singh, and Tiffani J. Johnson. 2017. A decade of studying implicit racial/ethnic bias in healthcare providers using the implicit association test. *Social Science and Medicine* 199: 219–229.

Marshall, Angela, and Kathy Palokoff. 2023. *Dismissed: Tackling the biases that undermine our health care.* New York: Citadel Press.

Meghani, S.H., Eeeseung Byun, and Rollin M. Gallagher. 2012. Time to take stock: A meta-analysis and systematic review of analgesic treatment disparities for pain in the United States. *Pain Medicine* 13 (2): 150–174.

Metzl, J.M., J. Petty, and O.V. Olowojoba. 2017. Using a structural competency framework to teach structural racism in pre-health education. *Social Science and Medicine* 199: 189–201.

Morra, Chiara. 2018. Black patients miss out on promising cancer drugs. *ProPublica.*https://www.propublica.org/article/black-patients-miss-out-on-promising-cancer-drugs. Accessed 6 June 2021.

Peek, N., J.H. Holmes, and J. Sun. 2014. Technical challenges for big data in biomedicine and health: Data sources, infrastructure, and analytics. *Yearbook of Medical Informatics* 9 (1): 42–47.

Project Implicit. 2021. About the IAT. https://implicit.harvard.edu/implicit/aboutus.html. Accessed 04 March 2021.

Sabon, J.A., and Anthony G. Greenwald. 2012. The influence of implicit bias on treatment recommendations for 4 common pediatric conditions: Pain, urinary tract infection, attention deficit hyperactivity disorder, and asthma. *American Journal of Public Health* 102 (5): 988–995.

Scharff, Darcell P., Kathleen J. Mathews, Pamela Jackson, Jonathan Hoffsuemmer, Emeobong Martin, and Dorothy Edwards. 2010. More than Tuskegee: understanding mistrust about research participation. *Journal of Health Care for the Poor and Underserved* 21 (3): 879–897.

Schulman, Kevin A., Jesse A. Berlin, William Harless, Jon F. Kerner, Shyrl Sistrunk, Bernard J. Gersh, Ross Dubé, Christopher K. Taleghani, Jennifer E. Burke, Sankey Williams, John M. Eisenberg, and José J. Escarce. 1999. The effect of race and sex on physicians' recommendations for cardiac catheterization. *The New England Journal of Medicine* 340: 618–626.

Sereno, Michelle, Jennifer Quigley, and Gregory S. Smit. 2021. A systematic review of the use of the implicit relational assessment procedure to assess implicit biases held by professionals toward client populations. *Research on Social Work Practice* 32 (1): 73–91. https://doi.org/10.1177/10497315211009.

Shirey, Theresa, and Alanna A. Morris. 2019. Different lenses for the same story: Examining how implicit bias can lead us to different clinical decisions for the "same" patient. *Journal of the American Heart Association* 8 (22): e014355.

Tamayo-Sarver, J.H., S.W. Hinze, R.K. Cydulka, and D.W. Baker. 2003. Racial and ethnic disparities in emergency department analgesic prescription. *American Journal of Public Health* 93 (12): 2067–2073.

Thomas, B., and Amber N. Booth-McCoy. 2020. Blackface, implicit bias, and the informal curriculum: Shaping the healthcare workforce, and improving health. *Journal of the National Medical Association.* 112 (5): 533–540.

U.S. Department of Health and Human Services. Agency for Healthcare Research and Quality. 2020. National healthcare quality and disparities report introduction and methods. https://www.ahrq.gov/research/findings/nhqrdr/nhqdr19/index.html. Accessed 5 Aug 2023.

U.S. Food and Drug Administration. 1998. Investigational new drug applications and new drug applications. https://www.fda.gov/ScienceResearch/SpecialTopics/RunningClinicalTrials/ucm120254.htm. Accessed 6 Aug 2023.

U.S. Food and Drug Administration. 2013. Collection, analysis, and availability of demographic subgroup data for FDA-approved medical products. https://www.fda.gov/media/86561/download. Accessed 6 Aug 2023.

U.S. Food and Drug Administration. 2014. Action plan to enhance the collection and availability of demographic subgroup data. https://www.fda.gov/downloads/regulatoryinformation/lawsenforcedbyfda/significantamendmentstothefdcact/fdasia/ucm410474.pdf. Accessed 6 Aug 2023.

U.S. Food and Drug Administration. 2016. Collection of race and ethnicity data in clinical trials: Guidance for industry and Food and Drug Administration staff. https://www.fda.gov/downloads/regulatoryinformation/guidances/ucm126396.pdf Accessed 6 June 2021.

U.S. Food and Drug Administration. 2017. Evaluation and reporting of age-, race-, and ethnicity: specific data in medical device clinical studies. https://www.fda.gov/downloads/MedicalDevices/DeviceRegulationandGuidance/GuidanceDocuments/UCM507278.pdf. Accessed 6 June 2021.

U.S. Food and Drug Administration. 2022. Diversity plans to improve enrollment of participants from underrepresented racial and ethnic population in clinical trials. Guidance for industry. https://www.fda.gov/media/157635/download. Accessed 20 June 2023.

U.S. Food and Drug Administration. 2019. Premarket approval (PMA). https://www.fda.gov/medical-devices/premarket-submissions/premarket-approval-pma. Accessed 6 June 2021.

U.S. Food and Drug Administration. 2020. Enhancing the diversity of clinical trial populations: eligibility criteria, enrollment practices, and trial designs. Guidance for industry. https://www.fda.gov/media/127712/download. Accessed 20 June 2023.

van Ryn, M., and Jane Burke. 2000. The effect of patient race and socio-economic status on physicians' perceptions of patients. *Social Science and Medicine* 50 (6): 813–828.

Warren, Rueben C., Lachlan Forrow, Davis Augustin Hodge, and Robert D. Truog. 2020. Trustworthiness before trust: Covid-19 vaccine trials and the black community. *New England Journal of Medicine* 383: e121.

Wendler, David, Raynard Kington, Jennifer Madans, Gretchen Van Wye, Heidi Christ-Schmidt, Laura A. Pratt, Otis W. Brawley, Cary P. Gross, and Ezekiel Emanuel. 2006. Are racial and ethnic minorities less willing to participate in health research? *PLoS Medicine* 3 (2): e19.

Zhang, Xinzhi, Eliseo Pérez-Stable, Philip E. Bourne, O. Emmanuel Peprah, Kenrik Duru, Nancy Breen, David Berrigan, Fred Wood, James S. Jackson, David W.S.. Wong, and Joshua Denny. 2017. Big data science: Opportunities and challenges to address minority health and health disparities in the 21st century. *Ethnicity and Disease* 27 (2): 95–106.

Chapter 5
Will Artificial Intelligence Improve Health Disparities?

Abstract The rapid pace of innovation is astounding, but it is also unsettling. Artificial intelligence holds great promise to improve health care, but the technology suffers with issues of biased data. Therefore, its usefulness as an instrument to reduce health disparities and improve the health of racial and ethnic minority groups is questionable. Implicit bias, explicit bias, missing data, and the lack of representation and diversity in datasets impact the data utility. Health disparities predate algorithms in health care. Its historical footprints are embedded into the data. Rather than being a panacea, algorithmic outcomes may exacerbate health disparities if biases in the data are not sufficiently addressed. Section 5.1 discusses the use of artificial intelligence to improve health disparities. Section 5.2 discusses principles and frameworks for ethical artificial intelligence. Section 5.3 proposes an algorithmic compliance framework to promote adoption of ethical artificial intelligence principles. Section 5.4 provides a summary of key points.

Keywords Disparities · Artificial intelligence · Transparency · Accountability · Inclusion · Compliance

5.1 The Use of Artificial Intelligence to Improve Health Disparities

Algorithms are common in health care. They are used in clinical care, health research, drug development, health systems management, public health surveillance, and diagnostic tools. As of October 2022, the U.S. Food and Drug Administration (FDA) listed 521 *artificial intelligence and machine learning (AI/ML) enabled medical devices* marketed in the United States (U.S. Food and Drug Administration 2022a). The list was not exhaustive, and inclusion was based upon publicly available information on AI/ML-enabled devices (U.S. Food and Drug Administration 2022a). Most of the devices were in the field of radiology, but others included cardiovascular, dental, clinical chemistry, ophthalmology, hematology, gastroenterology and urology, general and plastic surgery, microbiology, and pathology (U.S. Food and

N. H. Williams, *Artificial Intelligence and Healthcare*, The International Library of Bioethics 107, https://doi.org/10.1007/978-3-031-48262-5_5

Drug Administration 2022a). Some devices detected diabetic retinopathy, managed blood glucose, and analyzed radiology images for cancerous tumors. AI has the potential to improve health care and health disparities. For example, researchers discovered new subtypes of multiple sclerosis by using unsupervised machine learning to identify patterns in magnetic resonance imaging brain scans of people with the disease (Eshaghi et al. 2021). This discovery may help to develop new treatment approaches for multiple sclerosis. Other researchers developed models to predict suicide risk using real-time electronic health records (Walsh et al. 2021). These are just a few examples of its use in health care, but it is undeniable that AI may at least be an additional tool in the health care provider's arsenal to diagnose illness, increase treatment options, and improve treatment outcomes.

On the other hand, the use of an algorithm in medicine may be unnecessary to predict clinical significance. For example, researchers developed three machine learning models to predict in-hospital deaths for patients hospitalized for acute myocardial infarction (Khera et al. 2021). These models were compared to results from a logistical regression model, which is a standard statistical method. The study data included patient medical histories, demographics, comorbidities, medications, and laboratory test results. The researchers found the machine learning models were not clinically useful in predicting the risk of in-hospital mortality after acute myocardial infarction; they were equivalent to the logistical regression models results (Khera et al. 2021). This study demonstrates that algorithms do not always need to be the methodological technique of choice where traditional statistical methods will suffice.

Despite challenges with algorithmic bias, there is an argument to be made that AI may improve health disparities. In the United States in 2023, colorectal cancer represented 7.8% of all new cancer cases, preceded by breast cancer, prostate cancer, and lung and bronchus cancer (U.S. Department of Health and Human Services. National Cancer Institute. Surveillance, Epidemiology, and End Results Program 2023a). There will be an estimated 153,020 new cases and 52,550 estimated deaths (U.S. Department of Health and Human Services. National Cancer Institute. Surveillance, Epidemiology, and End Results Program 2023a). Colorectal cancer occurs in the colon or rectum where polyps (i.e., abnormal growths) can develop (U.S. Department of Health and Human Services. Centers for Disease Control and Prevention. Division of Cancer Prevention and Control 2023c). It disproportionately affects racial and ethnic minority groups (U.S. Department of Health and Human Services. National Cancer Institute. Surveillance, Epidemiology, and End Results Program 2023a). Between 2016 and 2020, the rate of new cases per 100,000 by race and ethnicity was as follows for both men and women: American Indian/Alaska Native (males 52.3/females 45.1); Black (males 50.4/females 37.2), White (males 42.3/females 32.5), Hispanics (males 39.6/females 28.4), and Asians/Pacific Islander (males 35.3/females 25.0) (U.S. Department of Health and Human Services. National Cancer Institute. Surveillance, Epidemiology, and End Results Program 2023a). Additionally, Black men, along with Black women and American Indian/Alaska

Native women, have the highest death rate from colorectal cancer than other groups[1] (Augustus and Ellis 2018; US Department of Health and Human Services National Cancer Institute 2023a). A colonoscopy is a screening test for colorectal cancer to identify precancerous growths (U.S. Department of Health and Human Services. Centers for Disease Control and Prevention 2023a). A physician inserts a thin tube into the rectum to look for polyps and cancer in the rectum and colon (U.S. Department of Health and Human Services. Centers for Disease Control and Prevention. Division of Cancer Prevention and Control 2023c). In 2021, the FDA approved the first machine learning device to help physicians identify cancerous lesions in real-time during a colonoscopy (U.S. Food and Drug Administration 2021). It is "composed of hardware and software designed to highlight portions of the colon where the device detects a potential lesion. The software uses artificial intelligence algorithm techniques to identify regions of interest. During a colonoscopy, the system generates markers, which look like green squares and are accompanied by a short, low-volume sound, and superimposes them on the video from the endoscope camera when it identifies a potential lesion." (U.S. Food and Drug Administration 2021). The device signals to the physician that additional investigation is necessary. This may include detailed visual inspection, tissue biopsy, or tissue removal (U.S. Food and Drug Administration 2021). Colorectal cancer screening improves morbidity and mortality outcomes because it identifies precancerous tissue before it becomes cancerous (U.S. Department of Health and Human Services. Centers for Disease Control and Prevention. Division of Cancer Prevention and Control 2023c). Consequently, if an algorithm-driven device can improve the screening and diagnosis of colorectal cancer, it has the potential to improve colorectal cancer disparities for racial and ethnic minority populations by identifying precancerous tissue early.

5.1.1 Examples of Artificial Intelligence Use in Health Care

The diagnosis of childhood asthma is another area where AI may improve health disparities. Asthma is a chronic lung condition that can restrict the airways (U.S. Department of Health and Human Services. Centers for Disease Control and Prevention 2019). In 2021, there were over 4.6 million children under the age of 18 with asthma in the United States (U.S. Department of Health and Human Services. Centers for Disease Control and Prevention 2023d). Over 1.8 million children had one or more asthma attacks within the last 12 months (U.S. Department of Health and Human Services. Centers for Disease Control and Prevention 2023d). From 2019 to 2021, the prevalence of asthma was highest in Black children (11.6%), followed by American Indian/Alaska Native (9.2%), Hispanic (5.9%), White (5.5%), and Asian (3.3%) children (U.S. Department of Health and Human Services. Centers for Disease Control

[1] Blacks (males 22.3/females 14.3); American Indians/Alaska Natives (males 20.8/females 14.3); Whites (males 15.5/females 11.1); Hispanics (males 13.5/females 8.5); and Asians/Pacific Islanders (males 10.9/females 7.7).

and Prevention 2023d). In 2020, over 270,000 children visited the emergency department due to asthma, and approximately 27,000 were hospitalized (U.S. Department of Health and Human Services. Centers for Disease Control and Prevention 2023d). The diagnosis of childhood asthma is important for disease management and treatment. Controlling asthma attacks results in fewer emergency room visits, hospitalizations, and school absenteeism (U.S. Department of Health and Human Services. Centers for Disease Control and Prevention 2019). Researchers discovered that machine learning models could be trained using electronic health records to predict which children, diagnosed with asthma before 5 years old, would continue to have persistent asthma (Bose et al. 2021). In another study, researchers developed a screening algorithm to prioritize students at high risk for asthma for school nurse outreach (Rabner et al. 2020).

Among women, breast cancer is the second most common in the United States (U.S. Department of Health and Human Services. Centers for Disease Control and Prevention 2023b). In 2020, White women had a higher new breast cancer rates per 100,000 (125.3) compared to Black women (119.6),[2] but the rate of cancer deaths was higher in Black women (26.4) when compared to all other racial and ethnic groups[3] (U.S. Department of Health and Human Services. Centers for Disease Control and Prevention and National Cancer Institute. U.S. Cancer Statistics Working Group 2023). Mammography screening, which is a low dose x-ray of the breast, reduces breast cancer deaths because it identifies cancer in the early stages of development (U.S. Food and Drug Administration 2022b). Researchers created a deep learning model to predict breast cancer risk. Specifically, the model predicted if a patient would develop breast cancer within 5 years of examination (Yala et al. 2019).

The algorithm used full-field mammography images to assess this risk (Yala et al. 2019). Full-field mammography, also known as digital mammography, replaces the x-ray film with "solid-state detectors, similar to those found in digital cameras, which convert x-rays into electrical signals. The electrical signals are used to produce images of the breast that can be seen on a computer screen or printed on special films to look like screen-film mammograms." (U.S. Food and Drug Administration 2022c). In the study, three models were developed—a full-mammography image-only model based on deep learning, a logistical regression model using breast cancer risk factors only, and a hybrid model that combined full-mammography images with breast cancer risk factors (Yala et al. 2019). Some of the risk factors included breast density, age, weight, menopausal status, and family cancer history (Yala et al. 2019). The results were compared to the Tyrer-Cuzick model, a traditional risk prediction method for breast cancer (Himes et al. 2016; Yala et al. 2019). The researchers found that the hybrid model was more accurate in predicting risk in both White and Black women than the Tyrer-Cuzick model (Yala et al. 2019). In addition, the hybrid model performed especially well for Black women. The image-only deep learning

[2] Rate of new cancers by race and ethnicity: White (125.3), Black (119.6), Asian and Pacific Islander (94.3), American Indian and Alaska Native (91.6), Hispanic (88.2).

[3] Rate of cancer death by race and ethnicity: Black (26.4), White (19.3), American Indian and Alaska Native (13.5), Hispanic (13.2), and Asian and Pacific Islander (11.5).

model also exceeded the Tyrer-Cuzick model (Yala et al. 2019). The researchers suggested that the deep learning image-only model could help patients who did not know their family medical histories, and it could be quickly implemented for breast cancer screening (Yala et al. 2019). In this instance, a screening tool with improved identification of breast cancer in women, especially Black women, has the potential to improve cancer health disparities.

In 2021, 38.4 million people in the United States had diabetes, about 11.6% of the U.S. population (U.S. Department of Health and Human Services. Centers for Disease Control and Prevention 2022a). Of those, 29.4 million adults aged 18 years or older were diagnosed with diabetes, while another 8.7 million were undiagnosed (i.e., unaware or did not report) (U.S. Department of Health and Human Services. Centers for Disease Control and Prevention 2022a). Diabetes was the eighth leading cause of death (U.S. Department of Health and Human Services. Centers for Disease Control and Prevention 2022a). Of those adults 18 years or older diagnosed with diabetes for 2019-2021, the prevalence was highest among American Indians and Alaska Natives (13.6%), Blacks (12.1%), Hispanics (11.7%), Asians (9.1%) and Whites (6.9%). Adults with education beyond high school had a lower prevalence of diagnosed diabetes (6.9%) compared to those with a high school education (9.1%) and those without (13.1%). The risk factors for diabetes-related complications include smoking, obesity, physical inactivity, high blood pressure, and high cholesterol (U.S. Department of Health and Human Services. Centers for Disease Control and Prevention 2022a). People with diabetes are at risk for vision loss and blindness from diabetic retinopathy, the most common eye condition for people with diabetes (U.S. Department of Health and Human Services. Centers for Disease Control and Prevention 2022a). Diabetic retinopathy damages the blood vessels around the retina, but early detection through a dilated eye exam and treatment can prevent vision loss. It is estimated that more than 800,000 Blacks have diabetic retinopathy, and that number may increase to over 1 million by 2030 (U.S. Department of Health and Human Services 2019). In 2018, the U.S. FDA announced the marketing of IDx-DR, the first medical device to detect greater than a mild level of diabetic retinopathy in adults with diabetes (U.S. Food and Drug Administration 2018). It was also the first device to be marketed that did not require a clinician to interpret the images or the results (U.S. Food and Drug Administration 2018).

> The device, called IDx-DR, is a software program that uses an artificial intelligence algorithm to analyze images of the eye taken with a retinal camera called the Topcon NW400. A doctor uploads the digital images of the patient's retinas to a cloud server on which IDx-DR software is installed. If the images are of sufficient quality, the software provides the doctor with one of two results: (1) more than mild diabetic retinopathy detected: refer to an eye care professional or (2) negative for more than mild diabetic retinopathy; rescreen in 12 months. If a positive result is detected, patients should see an eye care provider for further diagnostic evaluation and possible treatment as soon as possible. (U.S. Food and Drug Administration 2018)

This AI tool could reduce disparities in diabetic retinopathy, especially with the most impacted populations, by making screening more accessible and timelier because a clinician is not required to interpret the results (U.S. Food and Drug Administration 2018).

Similarly, there are disparities in pain management for racial and ethnic minority groups (Institute of Medicine 2011). Implicit bias and racial and ethnic stereotyping may play a role in physician-prescribing behavior (Institute of Medicine 2011). Pierson et al. used machine learning to predict patients' osteoarthritis knee pain using x-ray images, comparing it to standard radiographic measures like the Kellgren–Lawrence grade (KLG) (Pierson et al. 2021). The researchers also included the patients' perception of their pain in their analysis. They studied over 4172 patients, producing 36,369 observations (Pierson et al. 2021) and found that Black patients, lower income patients, and patients with lower education suffered from extreme pain. Pierson et al. trained a convolutional neural network to predict a pain score for each knee (Pierson et al. 2021). Particularly, when compared to the KLG method, the new algorithm accounted for 4.7 times more racial pain disparities, 2.0 times more income disparities, and 3.6 times more educational disparities (Pierson et al. 2021). The researchers concluded that standard radiographic measures of pain severity may ignore undiagnosed features (Pierson et al. 2021).

In short, the algorithm identified additional features that were not detected in severe osteoarthritis as defined by the traditional radiographic grading systems (Pierson et al. 2021). Consequently, patients who presented with severe pain but not with severe radiographic disease were overlooked for surgical interventions. The researchers' approach reduced unexplained disparities in knee pain. Equally important, the researchers concluded that the training dataset itself attributed to the reduction in disparities because the data were racially and socioeconomically diverse (Pierson et al. 2021). Moreover, the dataset linked the patients' pain perception with their outcomes (Pierson et al. 2021). This research can improve health disparities because it addresses disparities in pain diagnosis, management, and treatment. As discussed in the previous chapter, implicit bias may impact patient-physician interactions. By including patients' pain perception in the algorithmic analysis, this technology can supplement physician judgement, possibly circumventing implicit bias (Pierson et al. 2021).

Lastly, prostate cancer, the abnormal growth of cells in the male prostate gland, was the second most common cancer in the United States in 2023 (U.S. Department of Health and Human Services. Centers for Disease Control and Prevention 2022b, U.S. Department of Health and Human Services. Centers for Disease Control and Prevention 2022c, U.S. Department of Health and Human Services. National Cancer Institute. Surveillance, Epidemiology, and End Results Program 2023b). In 2023, there were approximately 288,000 new prostate cancer cases, which was 14.7% of all new cancer cases (U.S. Department of Health and Human Services. National Cancer Institute. Surveillance, Epidemiology, and End Results Program 2023b). Based on data from 2013-2019, the 5-year relative survival rate is 97.1% (U.S. Department of Health and Human Services. National Cancer Institute. Surveillance, Epidemiology, and End Results Program 2023b). Risk factors for prostate cancer include age, race, family history, and genetics (U.S. Department of Health and Human Services. National Cancer Institute 2022). Black men are more likely to get prostate cancer and more than twice as likely to die from it than other men (U.S. Department of Health and Human Services. Centers for Disease Control and Prevention 2022c). The death rate per 100,000 for Black men is 37.5, followed by American Indian/Alaska Native (19.5), White (17.8), Hispanic (15.3), and Asian/Pacific Islander (8.6)[4] men (U.S. Department of Health and Human Services. National Cancer Institute. Surveillance, Epidemiology, and End Results Program 2023b).

The two common methods to screen for prostate cancer are the prostate specific antigen (PSA) test and the digital rectal examination (U.S. Department of Health and Human Services. Centers for Disease Control and Prevention 2022d). The PSA test measures the level of PSA, a protein produced by both cancerous and non-cancerous tissue, in the blood. Generally, an elevated PSA may indicate cancer, but other factors such as age, race, an enlarged prostate, and prostate inflammation may explain an elevated PSA (U.S. Department of Health and Human Services. Centers for Disease Control and Prevention 2022d). PSA-based screening is associated with false positive results, which happens when there is an abnormal PSA, but the man does not have cancer. Many men experience anxiety from a false positive result (U.S. Department of Health and Human Services. Centers for Disease Control and Prevention 2022e). A subsequent biopsy is often performed to diagnose prostate cancer, which may cause complications such as bleeding, pain, and infection (U.S. Department of Health and Human Services. Centers for Disease Control and Prevention 2022e). Prostate cancer treatment includes surveillance and monitoring of the cancer, removal of the prostate, and radiation (U.S. Department of Health and Human Services. Centers for Disease Control and Prevention 2022e). Possible complications from treatment include incontinence, impotence, and bowel issues (U.S. Department of Health and Human Services. Centers for Disease Control and Prevention 2022e). Prostate cancer screening and treatment can lead to complications from prostate biopsies, overdiagnosis, and physiological harm (U.S. Department of Health and Human Services. Centers for Disease Control and Prevention 2022e).

In one study, researchers found that using artificial neuron networks led to improved prostate cancer detection and decreased PSA false positives, thereby preventing needless follow-up biopsies (Van Booven et al. 2021). For the patient, the decision to screen and ultimately pursue treatment requires an informed decision about the harms and benefits. This decision may be compounded by issues of implicit bias, access to quality care, and insurance status. If AI advances improve prostate cancer detection, it may be another tool that will help health disparity populations because trustworthy results (i.e. the decrease in PSA false positives), may improve the diagnosis, treatment, and management of prostate cancer. It may also build more trust in the test results because of the reduction of false positives.

As these examples demonstrate, AI may improve health disparities as another tool for early diagnosis, treatment, and disease management. While the technology itself may be helpful, a lack of availability and application may dampen its effectiveness for racial and ethnic minority populations due to issues like access to quality care and socioeconomic barriers to its utilization not only for patients but also for

---

[4] U.S. 2016–2020, Age-Adjusted.

medical practices and hospitals. For example, under-resourced hospitals or health care providers who treat underserved populations, some of which may be racial and ethnic minorities, may not have access to the new AI technology. Furthermore, patients may not have the financial resources to benefit from the technology. Lastly, apart from access and financial considerations, there is a knowledge gap about what AI is and its potential. Patient and provider education is necessary so that both can understand AI's role in diagnosis and treatment decisions. Patients should not only be informed if an AI tool is employed in diagnosis and treatment, but what the AI prediction means and how it is calculated. Patient and health care provider communication is key. The adoption of AI as a tool to improve health disparities not only depends upon eradicating algorithmic bias but addressing the socioeconomic contextual dynamics that may impede its adoption.

5.2 Principles and Frameworks for Ethical Artificial Intelligence

AI in health care is often called "black box" medicine because the decision-making process of the algorithm is often unknown (D'Antonoli 2020). Algorithmic techniques can be complex and use large amounts of data; consequently, it is difficult to explain how they work and derive their predictions. Often, algorithms are proprietary property, making it difficult to expose their inner workings (D'Antonoli 2020; Reddy et al. 2020). Algorithmic transparency involves revealing the algorithm's code and its data to the public (D'Antonoli 2020; Dragoni et al. 2020). Explainable AI is an attempt to make algorithms more transparent by illustrating their decision-making process in simple, understandable terms to humans (Dragoni et al. 2020). The ability to explain the algorithms' output and clinical decision-making process is essential. From the patient's viewpoint, knowing and understanding how the algorithm derives its recommendations builds trust and transparency, especially when making decisions about their health.

Ethical artificial intelligence is governed by a compilation of several principles, including accountability, trustworthiness, inclusion, privacy, safety, and fairness and justice, to name a few (Hagendorff 2020; Reddy et al. 2020). Accountability and trustworthiness in the adoption of AI tools are paramount. In the United States, the National Institute of Standards and Technology's (NIST) Artificial Intelligence Framework (AI RMF 1.0) identifies seven characteristics of trustworthiness in AI systems (U.S. Department of Commerce. National Institute of Standards and Technology 2023). They must be valid and reliable, perform as required and intended, safe so as not to endanger human life and property, secure and resilient to avoid, protect, respond, and recover from attack, accountable and transparent, explainable and interpretable, privacy-enhanced to safeguard "human autonomy, identity, and dignity" (U.S. Department of Commerce. National Institute of Standards and Technology 2023, p. 17) and fair by managing issues such as harmful bias and discrimination (U.S. Department of Commerce. National Institute of Standards and Technology 2023, p. 17).

Diakopoulos and Friedler (2016) described accountability as responsible reporting of algorithmic decision-making consisting of five components—responsibility, explainability, accuracy, auditability, and fairness. First, responsibility is the individual with the authority to respond to any adverse algorithmic effects. Second, explainability is an attempt to make algorithms more transparent by explaining their decision-making process in simple, understandable terms to humans (Diakopoulos and Friedler 2016; Dragoni et al. 2020). Third, accuracy identifies and benchmarks the source of the algorithm's data so errors can be mitigated (Diakopoulos and Friedler 2016). Fourth, auditability is the ability of non-developers to review the algorithm's behavior to ensure that it is behaving in a manner consistent with expectations (Diakopoulos and Friedler 2016). Lastly, fairness ensures that algorithms are not discriminatory or have a negative social impact (Diakopoulos and Friedler 2016).

The ability to replicate or reproduce scientific research results also confers trust and transparency on the algorithm's performance. Two approaches are to re-analyze the data using the same procedures and protocols and using different statistical methods to reach similar study results (The National Science Foundation and U.S. Department of Education 2018). It is "a minimum necessary condition for a finding to be believable and informative." (The National Science Foundation and U.S. Department of Education 2018, p. 1). In health care, reproducibility builds confidence and trust in the diagnostic results, especially when the technology is new. For example, researchers evaluated 511 machine learning conference papers from 2017 to 2019 based upon technical, statistical, and conceptual reproducibility (McDermott et al. 2021). They discovered that approximately 21% of the machine learning papers that focused on health care made their coding publicly available and approximately 55% utilized public datasets (McDermott et al. 2021). Furthermore, only 23% of the machine learning health care papers utilized multiple datasets to confirm their results (McDermott et al. 2021).

Likewise, Roberts et al. (2021) found that 85% of studies using machine learning to predict COVID-19 in chest radiological imaging failed reproducibility and quality checks. They identified 2212 machine learning research studies and analyzed 415 papers relevant to the use of machine learning to diagnose COVID-19 using radiological imaging (Roberts et al. 2021). Of the 415 papers, 62 were included in the systematic review. The researchers concluded that the studies lacked strong reproducibility and quality standards (Roberts et al. 2021). Many of the studies included: (1) biases from small datasets; (2) flawed methodology; (3) poor image resolution and quality; and (4) repackaged datasets that contained duplicate components. Moreover, the studies failed to match demographics across similar populations and injected implicit bias into the models by possibly including the most novel or serious cases (Roberts et al. 2021).

The lack of reproducibility in research erodes trust not only in the science but also the consumers' confidence in the technology. Reproducibility is vital for algorithmic applications, especially for those deployed in the health care environment because it may impact patient care, which can lead to poor diagnostic and treatment outcomes (McDermott et al. 2021). Reproducibility of results is especially important with racial and ethnic minority populations to instill trust that the AI-driven treatment recommendations or interventions are not random experimentation. As discussed in Chapter Three, historical trauma remains around experimentation and clinical trial abuses among racial and ethnic minorities. When examining whether artificial intelligence will improve health disparities, it is necessary that these issues are addressed.

AI ethical codes and frameworks have been discussed and produced by numerous organizations including governmental agencies, non-profits, for-profit entities, and researchers, to name a few (World Health Organization 2021). For example, in 2021, the World Health Organization identified six guiding ethical principles for artificial intelligence in health (World Health Organization 2021). The first is human autonomy, which includes understanding the role AI plays in decision-making, protecting privacy, and acquiring informed consent (World Health Organization 2021). Second, AI technology should protect human well-being and safety and the public interest, and it should do no mental or physical harm to humans (World Health Organization 2021). Third, AI systems should ensure transparency, explainability, and intelligibility so there is enough documentation on the design and use of the AI technology (World Health Organization 2021). Fourth, they should foster responsibility and accountability, which involves evaluating the AI technology during development and use, and the provision of redress for adverse effects (World Health Organization 2021). Fifth, AI technology should ensure inclusiveness and equity, safeguarding against bias being encoded into the system. Lastly, AI systems should be responsive and sustainable (World Health Organization 2021).

Likewise, the U.S. Food and Drug Administration, Health Canada, and the United Kingdom's Medicines and Healthcare Products Regulatory Agency developed ten guiding principles to promote safe artificial intelligence and machine learning technologies (U.S. Food and Drug Administration, Health Canada, and United Kingdom's Medicines and Healthcare Products Regulatory Agency (MHRA) 2021). The guiding principles for Good Machine Learning Practices for Medical Device Development are: (1) multi-disciplinary expertise is leveraged throughout the total product life cycle, which includes understanding the potential model's risks and benefits; (2) good software engineering and security practices are implemented that encompass risk management, data integrity, and data security; (3) clinical study participants and datasets are representative of the intended patient population, allowing for patient generalizability and bias management; (4) training datasets are independent of test datasets; (5) selected reference datasets are based upon best available methods ensuring the collection of clinically relevant data; (6) model design is tailored to the available data and reflects the intended use of the device; (7) the performance of the human-AI team is the focus; (8) testing demonstrates device performance during clinically relevant conditions; (9) users are provided clear, essential information, which includes the model's intended use, performance, data characteristics, and limitations; and (10) deployed models are monitored for performance and re-training risks are managed (U.S. Food and Drug Administration, Health Canada, and United Kingdom's Medicines and Healthcare Products Regulatory Agency (MHRA) 2021).

Badal et al. (2023) framework focuses on the AI researcher operating in the AI development process. Their eight principles incorporate health equity into the framework. For example, Principle 1 states the goal of AI tools should be to reduce health disparities. This principle includes ensuring that the AI tool is accessible and improves outcomes for the disparity population (Badal et al. 2023). The other principles are: (2) outcomes of AI tools should be clinically meaningful, enabling the clinician to evaluate the AI tool for risk, accuracy, and fairness; (3) AI tools should aim to reduce overdiagnosis and overtreatment; (4) AI tools should aspire to have high health care value and avoid diverting resources from higher-priority areas, thereby they should be financially viable for the medical institution, not increase patient costs, and increase benefit; (5) AI tools should consider the biographical drivers of health such as the individuals' lived experiences, including their socioeconomic and environmental conditions; (6) AI tools should be designed to be easily tailored to the local population because it would maximize precision by the algorithm being trained for a particular locale; (7) AI tools should promote a learning health care system, including monitoring and improvement; and (8) AI tools should facilitate shared decision-making (Badal et al. 2023).

Gebru et al. (2021) recommend creating datasheets for datasets to document machine learning, thereby providing transparency and accountability. These datasheets would document several aspects of the dataset such as its creation, strengths and weaknesses, proposed use, structure, and maintenance (Gebru et al. 2021). The datasheets are comprised of seven categories: motivation for dataset creation; dataset composition; data collection process; data preprocessing; uses; dataset distribution; and dataset maintenance (Gebru et al. 2021). Several questions incorporated into each category provide an opportunity for greater discussion around issues involving data (Gebru et al. 2021). For example, under the data collection process category, questions focus on how the data were collected, the timeframe of data collection, the ethical review process, and the sampling strategy if the dataset was a sample from a larger dataset (Gebru et al. 2021). The researchers note that there are implementation challenges, such as workflow modifications based upon organization infrastructure, incentivizing datasheet creation, and understanding the social, geographic, and historical dynamics when the datasets relate to people (Gebru et al. 2021).

Complementing datasheets for datasets, Mitchell et al. (2019) proposes the use of model cards to document the performance of human-focused machine learning models to standardize reporting and ethical fairness (Mitchell et al. 2019). The model card sections are not an all-inclusive list and may be modified according to the user and model. The sections may include: (1) model details such as the name of the developer, the model type and version, and information about the training algorithm; (2) its intended use such as the primary users and tasks; (3) factors such as distinct group categories that include cultural, demographic, and phenotypic characteristics, the tools used to capture model input, and the environmental conditions in which the model was deployed; (4) metrics like the reported performance measures and how the metrics are calculated; (5) evaluation data including the source and composition of the dataset, how it was processed, and the reason it was chosen; (6) information about the training data; (7) quantitative analysis, which includes model evaluation results; (8) ethical considerations, including potential risks and harms of the model and risk mitigation; and (9) caveats and recommendations, which may list further concerns not discussed (Mitchell et al. 2019). One of the goals of this framework is to give the user information about the machine learning model's limitations, including the types of errors that may occur (Mitchell et al. 2019).

Obermeyer et al. (2019) identified a racial bias in an algorithm used to predict the need for enrollment in health care management programs because the algorithm used health care costs as a proxy for health needs (Obermeyer et al. 2019). In that study, Blacks spent less on health care due to access barriers and discrimination, and therefore used less health care management programs compared to Whites (Obermeyer et al. 2019). It appeared that Whites needed additional health care services, despite the fact that Black patients were sicker (Obermeyer et al. 2019). The root of the problem was identified—a labeling error—and the algorithm was fixed to prevent a future occurrence (Obermeyer et al. 2019). As an outgrowth of their research on algorithmic bias, the researchers developed the Algorithmic Bias Playbook to help mitigate and diagnose bias in algorithms (Obermeyer et al. 2021). The researchers identified two categories of bias. The first occurs when the algorithm is trained on data that are not diverse (Obermeyer et al. 2021). The second category, referred to as label choice bias, occurs when the algorithm is predicting a biased proxy variable rather than the target it should be forecasting (Obermeyer et al. 2021). The Algorithmic Bias Playbook outlines a framework with four key steps: inventory the algorithms being developed and used by the organization; screen the algorithm for bias; retrain the algorithm by improving it or discontinuing its use; and set up processes to prevent future bias (Obermeyer et al. 2021). Similar to other frameworks, the researchers created an algorithmic bias sheet that breaks down each step into action items. For example, in Step 1, the development of an algorithm inventory includes talking with stakeholders about algorithm use and identifying a person to maintain the inventory (Obermeyer et al. 2021). Step 2, screening for bias, involves analyzing the algorithm to investigate what it is predicting (Obermeyer et al. 2021). Step 3, retraining the biased algorithm, attempts to retrain the algorithm but is use is discontinued if not retrainable (Obermeyer et al. 2021). Step 4 focuses on creating an environment of best practices to prevent future bias by establishing written policies and protocols; documenting the algorithm's bias risk, target outcome, training process and performance; and creating organization reporting systems where anyone can report concerns about the algorithmic bias without retaliation (Obermeyer et al. 2021).

Whereas the previous frameworks focused on transparency and accountability through documentation standardization and checklists, the National Institute of Standards and Technology's (NIST) Artificial Intelligence Framework (AI RMF 1.0) concentrates on risk management. The AI RMF 1.0 looks at the AI system "as an engineered or machine-based system that can, for a given set of objectives, generate outputs such as predictions, recommendations, or decisions influencing real or virtual environments. AI systems are designed to operate with varying levels of autonomy." (U.S. Department of Commerce. National Institute of Standards and Technology 2023, p. 1). Designed to address risk, the framework states that risk is the "composite measure of an event's probability of occurring and the magnitude or degree of the consequences of the corresponding event. The impacts, or consequences, of AI systems can be positive, negative, or both and can result in opportunities or threats. When considering the negative impact of a potential event, risk is a function of (1) the negative impact, or magnitude of harm, that would arise if the circumstance or event occurs, and (2) the likelihood of occurrence." (U.S. Department of Commerce. National Institute of Standards and Technology 2023, p. 4). The framework discusses how organizations may frame AI-related risk, and how organizations may manage risks through four core functions: (1) govern (i.e., cross-cutting implementation of a culture of risk management); (2) map (i.e., contextual analysis of the AI system impact); (3) measure (i.e., approaches to quantify, evaluate, and monitor risk); and (4) manage (i.e., resource allocation to risks that have been mapped and measured) (U.S. Department of Commerce. National Institute of Standards and Technology 2023). The framework serves a dual goal of minimizing the negative risk of AI systems while also identifying and maximizing the positive impacts (U.S. Department of Commerce. National Institute of Standards and Technology 2023). The intended use is to prioritize risk while allying with existing laws and regulations. In the AI RMF 1.0, the organization determines risk prioritization. It:

> may differ between AI systems that are designed or deployed to directly interact with humans as compared to AI systems that are not. Higher initial prioritization may be called for in settings where the AI system is trained on large datasets comprised of sensitive or protected data such as personally identifiable information, or where the outputs of the AI systems have direct or indirect impact on humans. AI systems designed to interact only with computational systems and trained on non-sensitive datasets (for example, data collected from the physical environment) may call for lower initial prioritization. Nonetheless, regularly assessing and prioritizing risk based on context remains important because non-human-facing AI systems can have downstream safety or social implications. (U.S. Department of Commerce. National Institute of Standards and Technology 2023, p. 8)

Risk management challenges include how third-party data and software are developed, deployed, and used by the consumer; the lack of methods to measure risk and trustworthiness; and the associated risks during the lifecycle of AI creation, deployment, and use (U.S. Department of Commerce. National Institute of Standards and Technology 2023). Other challenges include developing human baseline metrics for comparison, AI application in the real world versus a controlled environment, and the lack of transparency and documentation in AI development and deployment (U.S. Department of Commerce. National Institute of Standards and Technology 2023).

These guidelines and frameworks are helpful but are varied and utilize different approaches. Additionally, they are self-enforcement mechanisms and recommendations, but they do not have regulatory authority (Campolo et al. 2017; Hagendorff 2020). To ensure trustworthiness, accountability, transparency, and equity in AI tools, an enforcement framework is also necessary. These elements are vital so that AI can be a tool to improve health disparities. As discussed, and highlighted here, there are numerous frameworks that can be tailored for each organization to develop, implement, and deploy algorithms. However, their use is often voluntary, making implementation a challenge. Without the force of law or legal repercussions when an AI tool fails, it may be difficult to incentivize organizations to regularly incorporate these frameworks. One option would be to encourage organizations to be proactive in incorporating an AI framework when they create, implement, and deploy an artificial intelligence tool through a health care compliance framework.

5.3 Elements of an AI Compliance Framework

Traditionally, health care compliance programs ensure that health care organizations follow certain laws, guidance, and ethical standards within the industry. The goals of these programs include safeguarding patient health care information, privacy, safety, and quality care. They also promote risk management, quality assurance, research ethics, and compliance with laws that prevent fraud and abuse. If certain laws are violated, organizations and individuals can face penalties. The health care compliance programs are guardrails to protect against malfeasance, minimizing risk by creating a system of internal controls to monitor, audit, and report noncompliant activities (U.S. Department of Health and Human Services. Office of the Inspector General 1999, U.S. Department of Health and Human Services. Office of the Inspector General 2017). Such a framework may be applicable to AI governance. How do we incentivize companies to adopt an AI health care compliance approach? One strategy is to hold companies accountable and levy fines when their algorithms go rogue. For example, in 2023, New York City was the first jurisdiction in the United States to publish regulations on the use of AI-driven automated employment decision tools. Violations result in financial civil penalties. As more jurisdictions adopt such regulations, the incentive would be to create such programs for an organization's self-protection. Also, to build transparency and trust, companies may consider proactively having such programs to create goodwill with the communities that the algorithms serve, especially organizations that engage racial and ethnic minority populations.

In AI research, as with compliance programs, it is important to identify the root of the problem so it can be fixed to prevent future occurrences. Many of these frameworks attempt to do this by documenting the algorithm's creation, uses, data inputs, and health equity impacts. An effective compliance program "provides a mechanism that brings the public and private sectors together to reach mutual goals of reducing fraud and abuse, improving operational quality, improving the quality of health care services and reducing the cost of health care." (U.S. Department of Health and Human Services. Office of the Inspector General 1999, p. 36369). There are seven elements to a compliance program. These elements are: (1) implementing written policies, procedures, and standards of conduct; (2) oversight; (3) effective training and education; (4) developing effective lines of communication to report incidents; (5) conducting internal auditing and monitoring; (6) enforcing policies and taking disciplinary actions for violations; and (7) responding to detected offenses and undertaking corrective action (U.S. Department of Health and Human Services. Office of the Inspector General 1999, U.S. Department of Health and Human Services. Office of the Inspector General 2017). The seven elements alone do not determine compliance program effectiveness. Rather, effectiveness is measured by how the compliance program prevents and detects violations of the law, incorporates best practices, and minimizes risk (U.S. Department of Health and Human Services. Office of the Inspector General 1999, U.S. Department of Health and Human Services. Office of the Inspector General 2017). Applying this concept to algorithmic risk management, program effectiveness would be measured by how the compliance program prevents and detects algorithmic malfeasance, while incorporating best algorithmic practices and minimizing algorithmic harm to the public (Table 5.1).

Adapting the seven principles of an effective health care compliance program to an AI compliance framework incorporates elements from the guidelines and frameworks discussed in Sect. 5.2. Moreover, two additional elements are added. These are the

Table 5.1 Elements of a compliance program

Elements of a compliance program	Description
Implementing written policies, procedures, and standards of conduct	Implementation of understandable and consistent guidance to show how polices are implemented
Oversight	Must be a person of authority that oversees the general compliance program and must have direct access to the governing authority to notify them of issues
Effective training and education	Employees must be educated about the risk associated with their job function and the compliance program itself
Developing effective lines of communication	Establishing confidential channels where violations, events, or incidents can be reported
Conducting internal auditing and monitoring	Internal auditing to check the controls to make sure they are working as intended
Enforcing policies and taking disciplinary actions for violations	The policies must be applied consistently, and corrective action should be taken to avoid future incidents
Responding to detected offenses and undertaking corrective action	Identify the root of the problem (process, human, cultural) so that it can be fixed to prevent future occurrence

Adapted from: U.S. Department of Health and Human Services. Office of the Inspector General. 2017. *Measuring Compliance Program Effectiveness: A Resource Guide.* https://oig.hhs.gov/documents/toolkits/928/HCCA-OIG-Resource-Guide.pdf

management and elimination of bias in algorithms, and health disparities reduction, incorporating elements of the social determinants of health (Table 5.2).

When implementing written policies, procedures, and standards of conduct in the AI compliance framework, organizations should ensure that AI systems are transparent and explainable (World Health Organization 2021). This can be accomplished by creating and mandating polices that ensure that algorithms are cataloged, documented, monitored, evaluated, and their use explained (Gebru et al. 2021; Obermeyer et al. 2021). Oversight involves appointing a compliance officer and/or committee that is responsible for overseeing the integration of the compliance program into the organization, developing and implementing an annual compliance plan, and program and investigate any compliance violations (U.S. Department of Commerce. National Institute of Standards and Technology 2023). In this model, effective training and education not only promote an environment of compliance within the organization, but also provide accountability to patients. It involves internal organizational education on the regulatory policies as well educating the staff and consumers on algorithms, their use, and their impact in diagnosis, treatment, and care management (U.S. Food and Drug Administration, Health Canada, and United Kingdom's Medicines and Healthcare Products Regulatory Agency (MHRA) 2021). Developing effective methods of communication ensures that consumers are provided information about the algorithm's intended use, functioning, data characteristics, and limits (U.S. Food and Drug Administration, Health Canada, and United Kingdom's Medicines and Healthcare Products Regulatory Agency (MHRA) 2021). It also guarantees a feedback loop where both organization personnel and consumers can report algorithmic malfeasance without fear of retribution or concerns being disregarded. The next element, conducting internal auditing and monitoring, involves evaluating algorithms and the data they are trained on and evaluated with as well as documenting their performance (Mitchell et al. 2019). It also implements security practices and data integrity practices (U.S. Food and Drug Administration, Health Canada, and United Kingdom's Medicines and Healthcare Products Regulatory Agency (MHRA) 2021). Enforcing policies and taking disciplinary actions for violations entails organizations taking responsibility for evaluating algorithms during their development, implementation, and regular use, thereby providing remedies for their adverse effects (World Health Organization 2021). Within the organization, it also involves disciplinary actions for employees who may violate organizational AI compliance standards. Responding to detected offenses and undertaking corrective action means that AI tools should be retrained if they cause harm or no longer function under their intended use (Obermeyer et al. 2021). If the tools cannot be retrained, then they must be discarded (Obermeyer et al. 2021).

There are two additional elements added to the effective AI health care compliance program. These are bias management and elimination, and the reduction of health disparities. These elements can ensure that AI may be a tool to improve health disparities by prioritizing data inclusiveness, screening for biased algorithms, and reducing health disparities (Obermeyer et al. 2021; U.S. Food and Drug Administration, Health Canada, and United Kingdom's Medicines and Healthcare Products

Table 5.2 Elements of an AI health care compliance program

Elements of a compliance program	Action item
Implementing written policies, procedures, and standards of conduct	• AI systems should ensure transparency, explainability, and intelligibility so there is enough documentation on the design and use of the AI technology (World Health Organization 2021) • Datasheets would document several aspects of the dataset such as its creation, strengths and weaknesses, proposed use, structure, and maintenance (Gebru et al. 2021) • Inventory the algorithms being developed and used by the organization (Obermeyer et al. 2021)
Oversight	• Govern (i.e., cross-cutting implementation of a culture of risk management (U.S. Department of Commerce. National Institute of Standards and Technology 2023)
Effective training and education	• AI tools should promote a learning health care system, including monitoring and improvement (Badal et al. 2023)
Developing effective methods of communication	• Users are provided clear, essential information, which includes the model's intended use, performance, data characteristics, and limitations (U.S. Food and Drug Administration, Health Canada, and United Kingdom's Medicines and Healthcare Products Regulatory Agency (MHRA) 2021)
Conducting internal auditing and monitoring	• Good software engineering and security practices are implemented that encompasses risk management, data integrity, and data security (U.S. Food and Drug Administration, Health Canada, and United Kingdom's Medicines and Healthcare Products Regulatory Agency (MHRA) 2021) • Model cards to document the performance of human-focused machine learning models to standardize reporting and ethical fairness (Mitchell et al. 2019)
Enforcing policies and taking disciplinary actions for violations	• Foster responsibility and accountability, which involves evaluating the AI technology during development and use, and the provision of redress for adverse effects (World Health Organization 2021)
Responding to detected offenses and undertaking corrective action	• Retraining the algorithm by improving it or discontinuing its use; and setting up processes to prevent future bias (Obermeyer et al. 2021)

(continued)

Table 5.2 (continued)

Elements of a compliance program	Action item
Bias management and elimination	• AI technology should ensure inclusiveness and equity, safeguarding against bias being encoded into the system (World Health Organization 2021) • Clinical study participants and datasets are representative of the intended patient population, allowing for patient generalizability and bias management (U.S. Food and Drug Administration, Health Canada, and United Kingdom's Medicines and Healthcare Products Regulatory Agency (MHRA) 2021) • Deployed models are monitored for performance and re-training risks are managed (U.S. Food and Drug Administration, Health Canada, and United Kingdom's Medicines and Healthcare Products Regulatory Agency (MHRA) 2021) • Screening the algorithm for bias (Obermeyer et al. 2021) • Setting up processes to prevent future bias (Obermeyer et al. 2021)
Reduction of health disparities	• AI tools should consider the biographical drivers of health such as the individuals' lived experiences, including their socioeconomic and environmental conditions (Badal et al. 2023) • AI tools should be to used reduce health disparities (Badal et al. 2023)

Regulatory Agency (MHRA) 2021; World Health Organization 2021). The reduction of health disparities element incorporates the social determinants of health by including lived experience, socioeconomic, and environmental data (Badal et al. 2023).

There are several benefits to applying the health care compliance model to AI tools. First, it creates a system of monitoring and controls. Second, algorithm developers, coders, researchers, businesses, and other stakeholders in the AI ecosystem would understand that there will be zero tolerance for algorithms that purposely do harm, are biased, or not inclusive. Third, it communicates the organization's commitment to creating an environment of accountability. Lastly, it identifies a person of authority who responds to the violation and takes corrective action. The compliance model may not address all the issues associated with AI, but it provides a framework for enforcing the ethical ideals. It is the enforcement of AI ideals that will ensure that AI in health care benefits its consumers and eliminates data bias for racial and ethnic minority groups.

5.4 Summary

AI in health care holds great promise to improve health disparities. Its usefulness as an instrument to advance the health of racial and ethnic minority groups depends on whether the technology can overcome any bias embedded in the data. Some of the ethical AI frameworks and guidelines incorporate the drivers of these health disparities—the social determinants of health, structural racism, and implicit bias—by focusing on data inclusivity and equity. However, without formal regulation, organizations must adopt an enforcement mechanism for ethical AI, like an AI compliance model, to ensure the transparency, trust, and accountability of algorithmic systems.

References

Augustus, Gaius J., and Nathan A. Ellis. 2018. Colorectal cancer disparity in African Americans: Risk factors and carcinogenic mechanisms. *The American Journal of Pathology.* 188 (2): 291–303.

Badal, Kimberly, Carmen M. Lee, and Laura J. Esserman. 2023. Guiding principles for the responsible development of artificial intelligence tools for healthcare. *Communication in Medicine* 3 (1): 47.

Bose, Saurav, Chén. C. Kenyon, and Aaron J. Masino. 2021. Personalized prediction of early childhood asthma persistence: A machine learning approach. *PLoS ONE* 16: e0247784. https://doi.org/10.1371/journal.pone.0247784.

Campolo, Alex, Madelyn Sanfilippo, and Meredith Whittaker. 2017. AI Now 2017 report. https://ainowinstitute.org/publication/ai-now-2017-report-2. Accessed 11 Aug 2023.

D'Antonoli, Tugba Akiinci. 2020. Ethical considerations for artificial intelligence: An overview of the current radiology landscape. *Diagnostic and Interventional Radiology* 26 (5): 504–511.

Department of Commerce National Institute of Standards and Technology. 2023. *Artificial intelligence risk management framework (AI RMF 1.0).* https://nvlpubs.nist.gov/nistpubs/ai/NIST.AI.100-1.pdf. Accessed 15 July 2023.

Diakopoulos, Nicholas, and Sorelle Friedler. 2016. How to hold algorithms accountable. *MIT Technology Review.* https://www.technologyreview.com/2016/11/17/155957/how-to-hold-algorithms-accountable. Accessed 19 July 2023.

Dragoni, Mauro, Ivan Donadello, and Claudio Eccher. 2020. Explainable AI meets persuasiveness: Translating reason results into behavior change advice. *Artificial Intelligence in Medicine* 105: 101840. https://doi.org/10.1016/j.artmed.2020.101840.

Eshaghi, Arman, Alexantra L. Young, Peter A. Wijeratne, Ferran Prados, Douglas L. Arnold, Sridar Narayanan, Charles R.G.. Guttman, Frederik Barkhof, Daniel C. Alexander, Alan J. Thomson, Declan Chard, and Olga Ciccarelli. 2021. Identifying multiple sclerosis subtypes using unsupervised machine learning and MRI data. *Natural Communication* 12 (1): 2078. https://doi.org/10.1038/s41467-021-22265-2.

Gebru, Timnit, Jamie Morgenstern, Briana Vecchione, Jennifer Vaughan, Hanna Wallach, Ill Daumeé, and Kate Crawford. 2021. Datasheets for datasets. *Communications of the ACM.* 64 (12): 86–92. https://doi.org/10.1145/3458723.

Hagendorff, Thilo. 2020. The ethics of AI ethics: An evaluation of guidelines. *Minds and Machines.* 30: 99–120.

Himes, Deborah O., Aubri E. Root, Amanda Gammon, and Karlen E. Luthy. 2016. Breast cancer risk assessment: Calculating lifetime risk using the Tyrer-Cuzick model. *The Journal for Nurse Practitioners.* 12 (9): 581–592.

Institute of Medicine. 2011. *Relieving pain in America: A blueprint for transforming prevention, care, education, and research.* Washington, DC: National Academies Press.

Khera, Rohan, Julian Haimovich, Nathan C. Hurley, Robert McNamara, John Spertus, Nihar Desai, John S. Rumsfeld, Frederick A. Masoudi, Chenxi Huang, Sharon-Lise. Normand, Bobak J. Mortazavi, and Harlan M. Krumholz. 2021. Use of machine learning models to predict death after myocardial infarction. *JAMA Cardiology* 6 (6): 663–741.

McDermott, Matthew B.A., Shirly Wang, Nikki Marinsek, Rajesh Ranganath, Luca Foschini, and Marzyeh Ghassemi. 2021. Reproducibility in machine learning for health research: still a ways to go. *Science Translational Medicine.* 13 (586): eabb1655.

Mitchell, Margaret, Simone Wu, Andrew Zaldivar, Parker Barnes, Lucy Vasserman, Ben Hutchinson, Elena Spitzer, Inioluwa Deborah Raji, and Timnit Gebru. 2019. Model cards for model reporting. In *FAT* '19: proceedings of the conference on fairness, accountability, and transparency*, 220–229. https://doi.org/10.1145/3287560.3287596. Accessed 11 Aug 2023.

Obermeyer, Ziad, Brian Powers, Christine Vogeli, and Sendhil Mullainathan. 2019. Dissecting racial bias in an algorithm used to manage the health of populations. *Science* 366: 447–453.

Obermeyer, Ziad, Rebecca Nissan, Michael Stern, Stephanie Eaneff, Emily Joy Bembeneck, and Sendhil Mullainathan. 2021. Algorithmic bias playbook. https://www.chicagobooth.edu/-/media/project/chicago-booth/centers/caai/docs/algorithmic-bias-playbook-june-2021.pdf. Accessed 12 Aug 2023.

Pierson, Emma, David M. Cutler, Jure Leskovec, Sendhil Mullainathan, and Ziad Obermeyer. 2021. An algorithmic approach to reducing unexplained pain disparities in underserved populations. *Nature Medicine* 27: 136–140.

Rabner, Marc, Katherine Bissett, Sara B. Johnson, and Katherine A. Connor. 2020. A risk stratification algorithm for asthma identification and prioritization in a low-income urban school. *Journal of School Health.* 90 (7): 538–544.

Reddy, Sandeep, Sonia Allan, Simon Coghlan, and Paul Cooper. 2020. A governance model for the application of AI in health care. *Journal of the American Medical Informatics Association* 27 (3): 491–497.

Roberts, Michael, Derek Driggs, Matthew Thorpe, Julian Gilbey, Michael Yeung, Stephan Ursprung, Angelica I. Aviles-Rivero, Christian Etmann, Cathal McCague, Lucian Beer, Jonathan R. Weir-McCall, Zhongzhao Teng, Effrossyni Gkrania-Klotsas, James H. F. Rudd, Evis Sala, and Carola-Bibiane. Schönlieb. 2021. Common pitfalls and recommendations for using machine learning to detect and prognosticate for COVID-19 using chest radiographs and CT scans. *Nature Machine Intelligence* 3: 199–217.

The National Science Foundation and U.S. Department of Education. 2018. Companion guidelines on replication and reproducibility in education research. https://www.nsf.gov/pubs/2019/nsf19022/nsf19022.pdf. Accessed 11 Aug 2023.

U.S. Department of Health and Human Services. 2019. *National Eye Institute. African Americans with diabetes can prevent vision loss.* https://www.nei.nih.gov/sites/default/files/2019-06/african-americans-diabetes-can-prevent-vision-loss.pdf. Accessed 11 Aug 2023.

U.S. Department of Health and Human Services Centers for Disease Control and Prevention. 2019. *Asthma in children.* https://www.cdc.gov/vitalsigns/childhood-asthma/index.html. Accessed 18 July 2023.

U.S. Department of Health and Human Services. National Cancer Institute. 2022. *Prostate cancer prevention (PDQ®)–patient version.* https://www.cancer.gov/types/prostate/patient/prostate-prevention-pdq#section/all. Accessed 19 July 2023.

U.S. Department of Health and Human Services Centers for Disease Control and Prevention. 2022a. *National diabetes statistics report.* https://www.cdc.gov/diabetes/data/statistics-report/index.html. Accessed 18 July 2023.

U.S. Department of Health and Human Services Centers for Disease Control and Prevention. 2022b. *What is prostate cancer?* https://www.cdc.gov/cancer/prostate/basic_info/what-is-prostate-cancer.htm. Accessed 19 July 2023.

U.S. Department of Health and Human Services Centers for Disease Control and Prevention. 2022c. *Who is at risk for prostate cancer?* https://www.cdc.gov/cancer/prostate/basic_info/risk_factors.htm#:~:text=The%20most%20common%20risk%20factor,family%20history%20of%20prostate%20cancer. Accessed 19 July 2023.

U.S. Department of Health and Human Services Centers for Disease Control and Prevention. 2022d. *What is screening for prostate cancer risk?* https://www.cdc.gov/cancer/prostate/basic_info/screening.htm. Accessed 19 July 2023.

U.S. Department of Health and Human Services Centers for Disease Control and Prevention. 2022e. *What are the benefits and harms of screening?* https://www.cdc.gov/cancer/prostate/basic_info/benefits-harms.htm. Accessed 19 July 2023.

U.S. Department of Health and Human Services Centers for Disease Control and Prevention. 2023a. *Basic information about colorectal cancer*. https://www.cdc.gov/cancer/colorectal/basic_info/. Accessed 15 July 2023.

U.S. Department of Health and Human Services Centers for Disease Control and Prevention. 2023b. *Breast cancer statistics. https://www.cdc.gov/cancer/breast/statistics/index.htm.* Accessed 23 Sept 2023.

U.S. Department of Health and Human Services Centers for Disease Control and Prevention. Division of Cancer Prevention and Control. 2023c. *Colorectal cancer screening tests.* https://www.cdc.gov/cancer/colorectal/basic_info/screening/tests.htm. Accessed 15 July 2023.

U.S. Department of Health and Human Services Centers for Disease Control and Prevention. 2023d. *Most recent national asthma data. Current asthma prevalence by race and ethnicity (2019–2021).* https://www.cdc.gov/asthma/most_recent_national_asthma_data.htm. Accessed 15 July 2023.

U.S. Department of Health and Human Services Centers for Disease Control and Prevention and National Cancer Institute U.S. Cancer Statistics Working Group. 2023. *U.S. Cancer Statistics Data Visualizations Tool, based on 2022 submission data (1999–2020).* https://gis.cdc.gov/Cancer/USCS/?CDC_AA_refVal=https%3A%2F%2Fwww.cdc.gov%2Fcancer%2Fdataviz%2Findex.htm#/Demographics/. Accessed 23 September 2023.

U.S. Department of Health and Human Services National Cancer Institute. Surveillance, Epidemiology, and End Results Program. 2023a. *Cancer stat facts: colorectal cancer*. https://seer.cancer.gov/statfacts/html/colorect.html. Accessed 15 July 2023.

U.S. Department of Health and Human Services National Cancer Institute. Surveillance, Epidemiology, and End Results Program. 2023b. *Cancer state facts: Prostate cancer*. https://seer.cancer.gov/statfacts/html/prost.html. Accessed 19 July 2023.

U.S. Department of Health and Human Services Office of the Inspector General. 1999. Publication of OIG compliance program guidance for the durable, medical equipment, prosthetics, orthotics, and supply industry. *Off Inspector General.* 64(128) 36368–36389. https://oig.hhs.gov/authorities/docs/frdme.pdf. Accessed 11 August 2023.

U.S. Department of Health and Human Services Office of the Inspector General. 2017. *Measuring compliance program* effectiveness: a resource guide. https://oig.hhs.gov/documents/toolkits/928/HCCA-OIG-Resource-Guide.pdf. Accessed 11 Aug 2023.

U.S. Food and Drug Administration. 2018 FDA permits marketing of artificial intelligence-based device to detect certain diabetes-related eye problems. https://www.fda.gov/news-events/press-announcements/fda-permits-marketing-artificial-intelligence-based-device-detect-certain-diabetes-related-eye. Accessed 18 July 2023.

U.S. Food and Drug Administration. 2021 FDA authorizes marketing of first device that uses artificial intelligence to help detect potential signs of colon cancer. https://www.fda.gov/news-events/press-announcements/fda-authorizes-marketing-first-device-uses-artificial-intelligence-help-detect-potential-signs-colon. Accessed 15 July 2023.

U.S. Food and Drug Administration. 2022a. *Artificial intelligence and machine learning (AI/ML)-enabled medical devices.* https://www.fda.gov/medical-devices/software-medical-device-samd/artificial-intelligence-and-machine-learning-aiml-enabled-medical-devices. Accessed 18 July 2023.

U.S. Food and Drug Administration. 2022b. Mammographyi https://www.fda.gov/consumers/womens-health-topics/mammography. Accessed 18 July 2023.

U.S. Food and Drug Administration. 2022c. Frequently asked questions about digital mammography. https://www.fda.gov/radiation-emitting-products/consumer-information-mqsa/frequently-asked-questions-about-digital-mammography. Accessed 18 July 2023.

U.S. Food and Drug Administration, Health Canada, and United Kingdom's Medicines and Healthcare Products Regulatory Agency (MHRA). 2021. Good machine learning practice for medical device development: Guiding principles. https://www.fda.gov/media/153486/download. Accessed 12 Aug 2023.

Van Booven, Derek J., Manish Kuchakulla, Raghav Pai, Fabio S. Frech, Reshna Ramasahayam, Pritika Reddy, Madhumita Parmar, Ranjith Ramasamy, and Himanshu Arora. 2021. A systematic review of artificial intelligence in prostate cancer. *Research and Reports in Urology.* 13: 31–39.

Walsh, Colin G., Kevin B. Johnson, Michael Ripperger, Sarah Sperry, Joyce Harris, Nathaniel Clark, Elliot Fielstein, Laurie Novak, Katelyn Robinson, and William W. Stead. 2021. Prospective validation of an electronic health record–based, real-time suicide risk model. *JAMA Networking Open.* 2021;4(3): e211428.

World Health Organization. 2021. *Ethics and governance of artificial intelligence for health*: WHO guidance.

Yala, Adam, Constance Lehman, Tai Schuster, Tally Portnoi, and Regina Barzilay. 2019. A deep learning mammography-based model for improved breast cancer risk prediction. *Radiology* 292 (1): 60–66.

Chapter 6
Artificial Intelligence and Health Disparities: Policy, Regulation, and Implications

Abstract Industries and governments struggle to define artificial intelligence and regulate it to ensure that it is transparent, fair, and free of bias. This chapter discusses past and current regulatory proposals on artificial intelligence. Section 6.1 examines the artificial intelligence regulation debate. Section 6.2 focuses on the United States government's attempts to legislate artificial intelligence. Section 6.3 highlights the regulatory guidance from U.S. federal agencies. Section 6.4 provides an overview of the European Commission's landmark proposed legal framework to regulate artificial intelligence. Section 6.5 analyzes the impact of artificial intelligence regulation on health disparities. Finally, Sect. 6.6 summarizes key points in the chapter.

Keywords Artificial intelligence · Automated decision systems · Legislation · Regulation

6.1 Artificial Intelligence Regulation Debate

The artificial intelligence (AI) regulation discussion is multifaceted. With the wide use of generative AI applications like ChatGPT,[1] DALL-E,[2] and Bard[3] that produce various types of content, including audio, text, video, and images, the calls for AI regulation have become more urgent (Feingold 2023). An AI regulatory framework provides best practices on verifying, validating, and monitoring AI systems so they are fair, transparent, explainable, accountable, and diverse. Implementing and enforcing a regulatory framework can ultimately prevent biased and discriminatory impact (Diakopoulos and Friedler 2016; Fonzone and Heinzelman 2018). Proposed legislation to regulate AI incorporates many of the elements of ethical AI frameworks discussed in the previous chapter. These include requiring AI product

[1] https://openai.com/blog/chatgpt.

[2] https://openai.com/dall-e-2.

[3] https://bard.google.com/.

N. H. Williams, *Artificial Intelligence and Healthcare*, The International Library of Bioethics 107, https://doi.org/10.1007/978-3-031-48262-5_6

documentation, independent risk assessments, and new industry-specific rules. In the United States (U.S.), some entities have even proposed the creation of a new regulatory agency focused on AI (Lima and DiMolfetta 2023).

Regulatory proposals aim to guarantee efficacy, fairness, accountability, and transparency of AI systems, guarding against algorithms' use to perform nefarious acts, and building public trust and confidence in these systems (Char 2018; Hudson 2017). Critics of regulation argue that it will stifle innovation because the government does not have the technical expertise to legislate AI systems (Guihot et al. 2017). Moreover, the regulation would prolong the AI product development and deployment, inhibiting the field's growth (Bambauer 2017). Furthermore, data are dynamic and AI systems trained on data would need to be constantly updated and revalidated (Fig. 6.1).

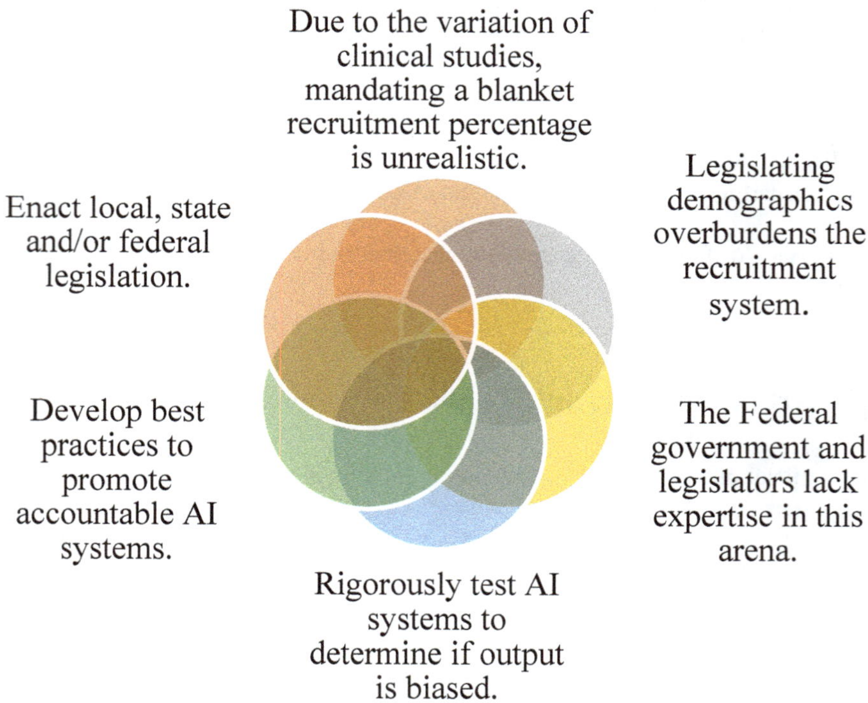

Fig. 6.1 The artificial intelligence regulation debate

Both critics and supporters of regulation share the common goal of protecting public safety and safeguarding against bias that may be built into algorithmic systems. To build confidence in AI systems and protect health disparity populations and racial and ethnic minorities in the United States, federal legislation is key as long as it safeguards against biased datasets; ensures that AI tools are evaluated for bias during development, deployment, and use; and infuses equity into the inception and development of AI systems. The development and use of AI systems demand that guardrails be put in place, not to impede the technology, but to allow it to grow and evolve in a responsible manner that protects society from its potential abuses.

The Volkswagen emissions algorithm (Greenemeier 2015) and the Uber Greyball (O'Neil 2017) algorithm are examples of algorithmic abuse. In 2015, the U.S. Environmental Protection Agency (EPA) determined that Volkswagen, a German automobile manufacturer, violated the Clean Air Act,[4] a U.S. federal law that regulates air emissions, because its emission control device used an algorithm to deceive emissions tests (U.S. Environmental Protection Agency 2015). Purposely, the device would detect when the car was undergoing emissions testing and then switch to a lower emissions setting (U.S. Environmental Protection Agency 2020). Roughly 11 million vehicles worldwide were affected. Consequently, the vehicles emitted excess pollution, including nitrogen oxide up to 40 times the normal level allowable in the United States (Hotton 2015). Moreover, researchers predicted that the excess emissions from affected cars sold in Germany between 2008 and 2015 would cause premature deaths in Europe (Chossière et al. 2017; Oldenkamp et al. 2016).

In another example of nefarious activity, Uber's Greyball algorithm was created to specifically allow its drivers to identify and evade authorities so they could operate illegally in cities worldwide (Isaac 2017; O'Neil 2017). Uber is an app and American technology company. The Greyball algorithm would identify regulatory officials or customers that violated Uber terms of service by using the data collected from the Uber app and other sources (Isaac 2017). This potential for algorithmic abuse is not limited to the automotive and technology industries. In the health care industry, the danger may arise from potential bias—either explicit, implicit, the lack of diversity in training databases, and incorrect outcome targets (Char 2018). In 2014, a U.S. White House report expressed concern about the discriminatory potential of AI (Executive Office of the President 2014).

> The technologies of automated decision-making are opaque and largely inaccessible to the average person. Yet they are assuming increasing importance and being used in contexts related to individuals' access to health, education, employment, credit, and goods and services. This combination of circumstances and technology raises difficult questions about how to ensure that discriminatory effects resulting from automated decision processes, whether intended or not, can be detected, measured, and redressed. We must begin a national conversation on big data, discrimination, and civil liberties." (Executive Office of the President 2014, p. 64).

The Volkswagen and Uber cases are early examples of why AI should be regulated, but the question remains how it should be done. In 2023, over 25 U.S. states, Puerto Rico, and the District of Columbia introduced legislation regulating artificial intelligence (National Conference of State Legislators 2023). Examples of state legislation include conducting a comprehensive inventory of all high-risk automated

[4] 42 U.S.C. §7401 et seq. (1970).

decision systems, minimizing the discriminatory impacts from automated decision systems, quantifying the negative mental health risks associated with social media and AI, identifying the use of race and zip codes in employment decisions where the employer uses data analytics, and mandating the study of the impact of artificial intelligence on laws, policies, and regulations (National Conference of State Legislators 2023). As an example, the state of Maryland prohibits employers from using "certain facial recognition services during an applicant's interview for employment unless the applicant consents."[5] Likewise, Illinois enacted the *Artificial Intelligence Video Interview Act*, which requires employers that use artificial intelligence in the interviewing process to notify the applicant in writing before the interview, provide the applicant with an information on how the technology works, and obtain consent, prior to the interview, to AI evaluation.[6] (Fitzgerald 2023).

In 2017, the New York City Council passed Local Law 49, considered the first law of its kind, creating a task force that would provide recommendations on the transparency of automated decision systems and how the city's agencies use the technology[7] (Richardson 2017). The New York City Automated Decision Systems Task Force (ADS Task Force) was established in 2018. The ADS Task Force's mandate was to provide specific recommendations "to address how New York City uses ADS, how ADS are managed, how information about them is retained, and what happens when the public asks about, or has a concern about, a specific ADS." (New York City 2019, p. 13). The ADS Task Force issued its report and recommendations in November 2019. The ADS Task Force's recommendations provided guidance on building infrastructure, procedural policies, transparency, and trust in AI systems. Its mandate did not focus specifically on regulating algorithms or datasets but rather building the foundation for a regulatory scheme (New York City 2019). Some of the ADS Tasks Force's recommendations included: establishing a centralized automated decision systems organizational structure, which incorporates fairness, transparency, innovation, efficiency, and accountability into its structure; creating best practices on ADS; educating the staff and public on ADS; and developing a risk assessment process to determine if ADS may disproportionately affect individuals or groups (New York City 2019, p. 13). Moreover, some of the recommendations included developing a procedure where people affected by a decision that was made with the assistance of or by an automated decision system can receive an explanation for the decision, implementing a procedure to determine if the agency's automated decision system has a disproportionate impact on certain populations, and incorporating fairness, transparency, accountability, and efficiency into the use and management of agency automated decision systems (New York City 2019, p. 13).

---

[5] Maryland House Bill 1202.Chapter 0446 (2020). Labor and Employment- Use of Facial Recognition Services—Prohibition https://mgaleg.maryland.gov/2020RS/Chapters_noln/CH_446_hb1202t.pdf.

[6] Artificial Intelligence Video Interview Act. Public Act 101-0260. https://www.ilga.gov/legislation/publicacts/fulltext.asp?Name=101-0260.

[7] New York City Council. Int. 1696–2017, N.Y. City Council. 2017. A local law in relation to automated decision systems used by agencies. http://legistar.council.nyc.gov/LegislationDetail.aspx?ID=3137815&GUID=437A6A6D-62E1-47E2-9C42-461253F9C6D0.

Continuing to lead in the AI regulatory area, in 2021 New York City passed Local Law 144, which focuses on automated employment decision tools.[8] Enforcement began in July 2023 (Lohr 2023). The law prohibits "employers and employment agencies from using an automated employment decision tool unless the tool has been subject to a bias audit within one year of the use of the tool, information about the bias audit is publicly available, and certain notices have been provided to employees or job candidates."[9] The new legislation provides definitions of key terms such as automated employment decision tool, bias audit, and machine learning. It also specifies the bias audit requirements, the data requirements, the requirements for the published results of the bias audit, and provision of notices by employers and employment agencies to employees and candidates for employment (Lohr 2023). The law requires companies that use AI automated employment decision tools to notify the applicants of its use, to audit the systems for bias annually, and be fined for violations (Lohr 2023). It also allows applicants to demand and be informed of the type of data being collected (Lohr 2023).

In the U.S., states have taken the lead in AI regulation, which may ultimately result in a patchwork of laws that differ from state to state, leading to inconsistencies in their application. Any enacted legislation, whether at the state or federal level, should not only focus on fairness, transparency, explainability, and accountability, but must also emphasize data diversity and representation to tackle algorithmic bias. This will safeguard equity for racial and ethnic minority populations and health disparity populations.

6.2 U.S. Government Federal Regulation of Artificial Intelligence

By 2021, nearly 70 countries adopted policies to address AI, including the United States (OECD.AI. 2021). For example, in 2020 the White House issued Executive Order (EO) 13,960, *Promoting the Use of Trustworthy Artificial Intelligence in the Federal Government* (Executive Order 13960 2020). Under the EO, U.S. government "agencies must therefore design, develop, acquire, and use AI in a manner that fosters public trust and confidence while protecting privacy, civil rights, civil liberties, and American values." (Executive Order 13960 2020, p. 78929). The EO also set forth guiding principles for the use of AI in government. AI must be lawful and

---

8 New York City Council. Int1894-2020. 2021. A local law in relation to automated decision systems used by agencies. https://legistar.council.nyc.gov/LegislationDetail.aspx?ID=4344524&GUID=B051915D-A9AC-451E-81F8-6596032FA3F9.

9 New York City Council. Int1894-2020. 2021. A local law in relation to automated decision systems used by agencies. https://legistar.council.nyc.gov/LegislationDetail.aspx?ID=4344524&GUID=B051915D-A9AC-451E-81F8-6596032FA3F9.

respectful; purposeful and performance-driven; accurate, reliable, and effective; safe, secure, and resilient; understandable; responsible and traceable; regularly monitored; transparent; and accountable (Executive Order 13960 2020).

Despite policy documents and executive orders, the United States has no formal federal law that expressly regulates AI. The approach has been to adapt existing laws and regulations, update those laws and regulations when needed, propose new regulatory schemes on the federal agency level, issue executive orders, and introduce legislation. For instance, in 2017, members of the U.S. Congress introduced a bipartisan bill to examine artificial intelligence and its impact on the workforce, education, and legal rights. The *Fundamentally Understanding the Usability and Realistic Evolution of Artificial Intelligence Act of 2017* tasked the U.S. Department of Commerce to lead government policy on AI (FUTURE of Artificial Intelligence Act of 2017).[10]

The legislation had several components. For instance, it required the establishment of a federal Advisory Committee to study AI development and implementation and advise the Secretary of Commerce on policy recommendations. Additionally, the legislation focused on workforce displacement due to AI, education in science and technology to prepare the workforce, and open sharing of data. Furthermore, the bill promoted collaboration on AI research and encouraged ethics training, government efficiency, and international cooperation and competitiveness around AI. Other sections addressed the issues of bias, accountability, ethics, and machine learning bias through the lens of cultural and social norms. Moreover, the bill focused on accountability and responsibility for AI systems that violate the law. The Advisory Committee mandate included studying the identification and elimination of bias "in the development of artificial intelligence and in the algorithms that support them, including with respect to the following: (1) the selection and processing of data used to train artificial intelligence; (2) diversity in the development of artificial intelligence; and (3) the ways and places the systems are deployed and the potential harmful outcomes." Additionally, the Advisory Committee was directed to study whether to "incorporate ethical standards into the development and implementation of artificial intelligence."[11] Lastly, the legislation studied the impact of AI on privacy rights and how the government can encourage the progress of AI to benefit all social and economic classes. The legislation did not pass in the U.S. Congress.

In 2019, the *Algorithmic Accountability Act*[12] was introduced in the U.S. Congress (Wyden 2019). The bill addressed bias at its root by mandating an automatic decision system impact assessment. The proposed legislation required companies that fell under this bill's purview to use independent auditors to conduct automated decision system impact assessments of new and existing high-risk automated decision systems, and data protection impact assessments of new and existing high-risk information systems. The automated decision system impact assessment evaluated the "automated decision system's development process, including the design and

[10] FUTURE of Artificial Intelligence Act of 2017, H.R. 4625, 115th Cong. (2017).

[11] See Footnote 10.

[12] Algorithmic Accountability Act of 2019, S. 1108, 116 Cong. (2019).

training data of the automated decision system, for impacts on accuracy, fairness, bias, discrimination, privacy, and security"[13] as well as the risks it may pose. The data protection impact assessment studied the degree to which the information system protected the privacy and security of personal information. It also required companies to remediate any discrimination and bias identified from the assessments. This legislation did not pass in the U.S. Congress either.

The William M. Thornberry National Defense Authorization Act of 2021 (NDAA), which authorizes the fiscal year 2021 appropriations for the U.S. Department of Defense, became law on January 21, 2021.[14] The NDAA contained comprehensive initiatives regarding AI, but it did not set forth specific rules to regulate algorithms. The non-Department of Defense AI provisions created the National Artificial Intelligence Initiative Office. The Office's mission is to be the interface for federal AI activities. This includes planning and coordinating federal AI research, conducting stakeholder outreach for input on AI initiatives, supporting AI research and development, and developing educational and workforce programs geared towards AI. Equally important, the law coordinates activities throughout the U.S. government to examine the ethical, legal, safety, privacy, and bias issues related to AI systems. It also addresses geographic disparities by examining how AI can improve opportunities in urban, rural, and Tribal communities. Lastly, the law encourages international collaboration on AI research, standards development, and regulation. The military provisions pertain to the acquisition of ethically and responsibly developed AI technology, establishing a steering committee on emerging technology, and developing AI standards (Stanford University 2021).

Apart from the NDAA, the United States is still developing a federal legislative AI strategy. In October 2022, the White House Office of Science Policy and Technology published the *Blueprint for an AI Bill of Rights*, which details five guiding principles for the design, use, and deployment of automated systems (The White House Office of Science and Technology Policy 2022). These principles are: (1) safe and effective systems, (2) algorithmic discrimination protections, (3) data privacy, notice and explanation, and (4) human alternatives, consideration, and fallback (The White House Office of Science and Technology Policy 2022). Edited excerpts from the AI Bill of Rights are listed in Table 6.1. It represents a framework that can serve as a foundation for legislative action. The first principle, safe and effective systems, focuses on protecting the public from harmful automated systems. Specifically, it endorses pre-deployment testing, identifying risk, monitoring, and mitigating risk. Equally important, if the system does not protect people from harm, it should not be deployed or should be removed completely (The White House Office of Science and Technology Policy 2022). Algorithmic discrimination occurs when "automated systems contribute to unjustified different treatment or impacts disfavoring people based on their race, color, ethnicity, sex (including pregnancy, childbirth, and related medical conditions, gender identity, intersex status, and sexual orientation), religion,

[13] Algorithmic Accountability Act of 2019, S. 1108, 116 Cong. (2019), 2.

[14] The National Defense Authorization Act of 2021. Pub. L. No. 116-28.

Table 6.1 Blueprint for an AI bill of rights

Excerpts from the Blueprint for an AI Bill of Rights	
Safe and effective systems	• "Automated systems should be developed with consultation from diverse communities, stakeholders, and domain experts to identify concerns, risks, and potential impacts of the system. • Systems should undergo pre-deployment testing, risk identification and mitigation, and ongoing monitoring. • Outcomes of these protective measures should include the possibility of not deploying the system or removing a system from use."
Algorithmic discrimination protections	• "Designers, developers, and deployers of automated systems should take proactive and continuous measures to protect individuals and communities from algorithmic discrimination and to use and design systems in an equitable way."
Data privacy	• "Designers, developers, and deployers of automated systems should seek permission and respect decisions regarding collection, use, access, transfer, and deletion of your data. • Consent should only be used to justify collection of data in cases where it can be appropriately and meaningfully given. • Any consent requests should be brief, be understandable in plain language, and give the person agency over data collection and the specific context of use. • Enhanced protections and restrictions for data and inferences related to sensitive domains, including health, work, education, criminal justice, and finance, and for data pertaining to youth. • Surveillance technologies should be subject to heightened oversight that includes at least pre-deployment assessment of their potential harms and scope limits to protect privacy and civil liberties."
Notice and explanation	• "Designers, developers, and deployers of automated systems should provide generally accessible plain language documentation. • Automated systems should provide explanations that are technically valid, meaningful and useful. • Reporting that includes summary information about these automated systems in plain language and assessments of the clarity and quality of the notice and explanations should be made public whenever possible."

(continued)

Table 6.1 (continued)

Human alternatives, consideration, and fallback	• "People should be able to opt out from automated systems in favor of a human alternative, where appropriate. • People should have access to timely human consideration and remedy by a fallback and escalation process if an automated system fails."

Source Blueprint for an AI Bill of Rights: Making Automated Systems Work for the American People. Office of Science and Technology Policy. https://www.whitehouse.gov/ostp/ai-bill-of-rights/

age, national origin, disability, veteran status, genetic information, or any other classification protected by law." (The White House Office of Science and Technology Policy 2022). The Blueprint urges creators of automated systems to be proactive in ensuring equitable design and protecting people from discrimination by conducting equity assessments, using representative data, and protecting against the use of proxy variables for demographic features (The White House Office of Science and Technology Policy 2022). Data privacy includes data protection, freedom from unchecked surveillance technologies, and obtaining consent (The White House Office of Science and Technology Policy 2022). This principle also carves out enhanced data protections and restrictions for health, work, education, criminal justice, and finance, and for data pertaining to youth (The White House Office of Science and Technology Policy 2022). For automated systems to be equitable, the Blueprint advocates for notices that document these systems in plain language and explains outcomes in a clear, timely, and accessible manner (The White House Office of Science and Technology Policy 2022). Lastly, the Blueprint requires human alternatives, consideration, and fallback. This means that people should have an alternative to using an AI system. Therefore, a human being should be available to respond in case the automated system fails (The White House Office of Science and Technology Policy 2022).

The goal to create a regulatory framework was endorsed by technology companies in the United States. In July 2023, U.S. President Joseph Biden secured voluntary commitments from seven AI companies—Amazon, Anthropic, Google, Inflection, Meta, Microsoft, and OpenAI—to encourage, safe, secure, and transparent development of AI technology (Bartz and Krystal 2023; Zakrzewski 2023). Specifically, the companies committed to ensuring safe products before public deployment, prioritizing security when creating AI systems, and building public support (Bartz and Krystal 2023; Zakrzewski 2023). In particular, the companies will permit independent experts to evaluate AI systems before deployment, share safety data on their systems, invest in cybersecurity, and watermark content that is AI generated (Bartz and Krystal 2023; Zakrzewski 2023). However, their commitment is not mandatory and does not include deadlines or reporting requirements (Zakrzewski 2023). The key focus areas are summarized in Table 6.2.

Table 6.2 FACT SHEET: Biden-Harris administration secures voluntary commitments from leading artificial intelligence companies to manage the risks posed by AI

<table>
<tr><td>Ensuring products are safe before introducing them to the public</td><td colspan="2">"The companies commit to internal and external security testing of their AI systems before their release. This testing, which will be carried out in part by independent experts, guards against some of the most significant sources of AI risks, such as biosecurity and cybersecurity, as well as its broader societal effects."</td><td colspan="2">"The companies commit to sharing information across the industry and with governments, civil society, and academia on managing AI risks. This includes best practices for safety, information on attempts to circumvent safeguards, and technical collaboration."</td></tr>
<tr><td>Building systems that put security first</td><td colspan="2">"The companies commit to investing in cybersecurity and insider threat safeguards to protect proprietary and unreleased model weights. These model weights are the most essential part of an AI system, and the companies agree that it is vital that the model weights be released only when intended and when security risks are considered."</td><td colspan="2">"The companies commit to facilitating third-party discovery and reporting of vulnerabilities in their AI systems. Some issues may persist even after an AI system is released and a robust reporting mechanism enables them to be found and fixed quickly."</td></tr>
<tr><td>Earning the public's trust</td><td>"The companies commit to developing robust technical mechanisms to ensure that users know when content is AI generated, such as a watermarking system. This action enables creativity with AI to flourish but reduces the dangers of fraud and deception."</td><td>"The companies commit to publicly reporting their AI systems' capabilities, limitations, and areas of appropriate and inappropriate use. This report will cover both security risks and societal risks, such as the effects on fairness and bias."</td><td>"The companies commit to prioritizing research on the societal risks that AI systems can pose, including on avoiding harmful bias and discrimination, and protecting privacy. The track record of AI shows the insidiousness and prevalence of these dangers, and the companies commit to rolling out AI that mitigates them."</td><td>"The companies commit to develop and deploy advanced AI systems to help address society's greatest challenges. From cancer prevention to mitigating climate change to so much in between, AI—if properly managed—can contribute enormously to the prosperity, equality, and security of all."</td></tr>
</table>

The White House. https://www.whitehouse.gov/briefing-room/statements-releases/2023/07/21/fact-sheet-biden-harris-administration-secures-voluntary-commitments-from-leading-artificial-intelligence-companies-to-manage-the-risks-posed-by-ai/

While these commitments and policy actions will move the discussion forward in cultivating AI systems that are fair, transparent, explainable, and accountable, none of them are mandated or enshrined in law (Bartz and Krystal 2023; Zakrzewski 2023).

6.3 U.S. Federal Trade Commission Guidance on Artificial Intelligence

Although the U.S. federal government has not enacted explicit legislation to regulate algorithms, there are existing U.S. laws that may be used to combat algorithmic bias. The U.S. Federal Trade Commission (FTC) is a government agency that protects consumers from unfair or deceptive acts or practices and promotes fair competition in the marketplace. It indirectly regulates algorithms through its consumer protection authorities (U.S. Federal Trade Commission 2016). In 2016, the FTC[15] issued its guidance, *Big Data: A Tool for Inclusion or Exclusion?* (U.S. Federal Trade Commission 2016). In that guidance, the FTC outlined several consumer protection laws that may be applicable in protecting the public against harm from AI systems and predictive analytics (Jillson 2021; Smith 2020). First, the Fair Credit Reporting Act (FCRA) pertains to "consumer reporting agencies that compile and sell consumer reports, which contain consumer information that is used or expected to be used for credit, employment, insurance, housing, or other similar decisions about consumers' eligibility for certain benefits and transactions." (U.S. Federal Trade Commission 2016, p. ii). In short, it regulates consumer reporting agencies that sell and assemble consumer reports. The FCRA applies when an algorithm denies people employment, housing, credit, insurance, or other benefits (Jillson 2021).

Second, the Federal Trade Commission Act (FTC Act) forbids unfair or deceptive acts or practices (U.S. Federal Trade Commission 2016). An act or practice "is deceptive if it involves a material statement or omission that is likely to mislead a consumer acting reasonably under the circumstances." (U.S. Federal Trade Commission 2016, p. 21). The FTC Act also applies if an act or practice is "likely to cause substantial consumer injury, the injury is not reasonably avoidable by consumers, and the injury is not outweighed by benefits to consumers or competition." (U.S. Federal Trade Commission 2016, p. 22). The FTC Act also applies to companies involved in big data analytics.

> Companies engaging in big data analytics should consider whether they are violating any material promises to consumers—whether that promise is to refrain from sharing data with third parties, to provide consumers with choices about sharing, or to safeguard consumers' personal information—or whether they have failed to disclose material information to consumers. In addition, companies that maintain big data on consumers should take care to reasonably secure consumers' data. Further, at a minimum, companies must not sell their big data analytics products to customers if they know or have reason to know that those customers will use the products for fraudulent or discriminatory purposes. The inquiry will

---

[15] The U.S. Federal Trade Commission enforces U.S. consumer protection laws.

> be fact-specific, and in every case, the test will be whether the company is offering or using big data analytics in a deceptive or unfair way. (US Federal Trade Commission 2016, p. iv).

Additionally, the FTC Act may apply if products sold to customers are used for discriminatory purposes, such as the sale and use of race-biased algorithms (Jillson 2021).

Lastly, the FTC enforces the Equal Credit Opportunity Act (ECOA), where "it is illegal for a company to use a biased algorithm that results in credit discrimination on the basis of race, color, religion, national origin, sex, marital status, age, or because a person receives public assistance." (Jillson 2021). To demonstrate a violation, the plaintiff must prove disparate treatment, which occurs when someone is treated differently based upon their race, color, religion, national origin, marital status, age, or receives public assistance (US Federal Trade Commission 2016). These are protected classes.

> Disparate impact analysis has important implications for big data. Under such an analysis, a company that avoids, for example, expressly screening job applicants based on gender and instead uses big data analytics to screen job applicants in a way that has a disparate impact on women may still be subject to specific equal employment opportunity laws, if the screening does not serve a legitimate business need or if the need can reasonably be achieved by another means with a smaller disparate impact. Likewise, if a company makes credit decisions based on zip codes, it may be violating ECOA if the decisions have a disparate impact on a protected class and are not justified by a legitimate business necessity. Even if evidence shows the decisions are justified by a business necessity, if there is a less discriminatory alternative, the decisions may still violate ECOA. (US Federal Trade Commission 2016, p. 19).

To prevent enforcement actions against companies, the FTC advises them to address gaps in data and algorithm model design, periodically monitor and test algorithms for discriminatory outcomes, be transparent and honest about how data are used, and be accountable for the algorithm's performance (Jillson 2021; U.S. Federal Trade Commission 2016).

The FTC Act is not designed to regulate AI specifically. Rather, it provides a source of action for those who are discriminated against, treated unfairly, or deceived by algorithms (Lima and DiMolfetta 2023).

6.4 The European Commission Proposed Legal Framework for Artificial Intelligence Regulation

In April 2021, the European Commission released its first European Union (EU) legal framework to regulate AI titled *Laying Down Harmonised Rules on Artificial Intelligence (Artificial Intelligence Act) and Amending Certain Union Legislative Acts* (European Commission 2021). The framework evaluates AI using a risk-based approach (European Parliament 2023). The first category is AI uses that pose an unacceptable risk. This prohibited category includes AI systems that: use subconscious techniques to affect an individual's behavior; classify individuals based on their social behavior or characteristics; and real-time biometric identification systems like facial recognition technologies (European Parliament 2023). There is an exception for remote biometric identification systems in the prosecution of serious crimes after approval (European Parliament 2023).

The second category in the legal framework is high-risk AI systems, which are systems that adversely affect safety and fundamental rights (European Parliament 2023). It is divided into two categories (European Parliament 2023). The first category is safety components of products such as toys, cars, aviation, medical devices, and equipment (European Parliament 2023). There are eight types of AI systems that fall under the second category (European Parliament 2023). These include AI systems used in (1) critical infrastructure management and operations; (2) education and vocational training and evaluation; (3) biometric identification systems; (4) employment, employee management, self-employment, and recruitment; (5) necessary public and private services; (6) law enforcement; (7) border control, migration, and asylum management; and (8) the administration of justice and democratic processes (European Parliament 2023). If a high-risk AI system is created, it must undergo an assessment process before placement on the market or service and throughout its lifetime (European Parliament 2023).

Limited risk AI systems require minimal transparency obligations, but users should be aware that they are talking with an AI system (European Parliament 2023). At that point, the user can decide whether or not to engage with the technology (European Parliament 2023). Likewise, minimal risk AI, which includes video games and spam filters, may have minimal transparency requirements (Feingold 2023). In June 2023, the most recent version of the proposed EU framework passed the European Parliament. Under this version, generative AI tools must comply with transparency requirements and there must be published summaries of copyrighted material used to train the system and safeguards from generating illegal content. The proposed law would establish the European Artificial Intelligence Board to develop AI standards, share best practices, and facilitate the implementation of the legal framework (Feingold 2023). With the adoption of amendments in June 2023, negotiation commenced with the EU member countries (Feingold 2023; Satariano 2023).

6.5 Implications for Health Disparities

The regulation of AI is a daunting challenge. Self-regulation will not be enough when balanced with the risks that AI presents. Many of the regulatory proposals discussed establish foundational frameworks that will create sustainable AI regulation. All incorporate the basic tenets of an ethical AI governance structure—fairness, trustworthiness, transparency, and accountability (Reddy et al. 2020). One recommendation would be to include public outreach and education in AI regulation.

One of the goals is to build public trust in AI systems. To do so, there must be public outreach and education to inform people about what AI actually is and its positive and negative impacts. It is crucial in the regulation of AI systems. Public opinion on AI spans a wide spectrum, ranging from being a helpful tool in medical diagnosis to posing as a threat to humanity. As an example, in a survey on Americans' perceptions of AI and the extent those perceptions are shaped by entertainment media, researchers found that people were more positive than negative about the technology. However, those who were more positive were White, male, younger, more educated, or lived in a populated area. Those who were more pessimistic were older, female, less educated, or lived in rural areas (Nader et al. 2022). In another survey, researchers found that most participants viewed AI in health care as beneficial but were less aware about its health applications, and they had concerns regarding decision-making applications and health information privacy (Beets et al. 2023). Therefore, any legislation should have a public outreach and education component to address the lack of knowledge about AI, its use, privacy concerns, and the public's rights in its creation, deployment, monitoring, and removal, if necessary.

Additionally, the legislative proposals do not focus directly on health disparities. They do address data bias and prioritize equity. They also recommend that systems undergo pre-deployment testing, risk identification and mitigation, and ongoing monitoring for bias and discriminatory effects. However, for AI to be a tool to improve health disparities, any legislative proposal must address how AI may or may not improve health disparities. One legislative proposal is to create a task force on algorithmic bias in health care. It would develop guidance to ensure that AI systems are created, deployed, integrated, and monitored to improve, not exacerbate, health disparities and are free from data bias.[16] To optimize AI as a tool to reduce health disparities, legislation should incorporate the following recommendations:

1. Integrate standardized demographic information and social determinants into data and link geographic variables and social determinants to clinical data.
2. Increase the participation of racial and ethnic minorities in clinical trials to improve data diversity and inclusiveness.
3. In studies with limited racial and ethnic minority data, examine how AI computational techniques may be used to impute missing data.
4. Develop and fund research that examines whether data bias reduces or increases disparities in health and health care.
5. Fund research on the use of AI as a tool to reduce health disparities.
6. Develop policies and regulations that mandate a specific percentage of racial and ethnic minorities be included in drug and device studies that reflect the prevalence of the disease condition in the population.
7. Create a data inclusivity report card that grades databases based upon the inclusion of racial and ethnic minorities, standardized demographic information, and the social determinants of health.
8. Provide outreach and education to the public on AI, its strengths and weak-

[16] Health Equity and Accountability Act of 2022, H.R. 7585. 117 Cong. (2022).

nesses, and possible impact.

9. Diversify the biomedical and technology workforce so that the ideas, perceptions, and values of racial and ethnic minority groups are represented in the creation, deployment, and evaluation of AI tools.
10. Incorporate penalties into a regulatory framework for companies that create AI tools that do harm the public, as well as provide redress for those that are harmed.

AI regulation is a balance of risks. The challenge is to create legislation that does not stifle innovation but ensures equity as well as fairness and justice, safety, accountability, trustworthiness, and transparency. Any legislation must also safeguard against bias that may be built into algorithmic systems, but also removes those systems if they cause harm and cannot be retrained. For AI to improve health disparities, equity, diversity, and representation must be incorporated in the development, deployment, and evaluation of these systems as well as the data on which these systems are trained.

6.6 Summary

There is an urgency to regulate AI. Both critics and supporters of regulation share the common goal of protecting public safety and safeguarding against bias that may be built into algorithmic systems. Implementing and enforcing a regulatory framework can ultimately prevent biased and discriminatory impact. Any regulation should also punish unscrupulous AI actors. In the U.S, the states have taken the lead in AI regulation, but the federal government is invested in developing a comprehensive AI legislation that is equitable and fair. After years of formulation, the European Union is on the verge of passing a law to regulate AI based upon risk. To ensure that AI does not exacerbate disparities, any legislative proposals must tackle algorithmic bias in all its forms during the creation, deployment, and evaluation of AI systems.

References

Bambauer, Jane R. 2017. Dr. Robot. 51 U.C. Davis L. Review 51(383): 385–398.

Bartz, Diane, and Krystal Hu. 2023. OpenAI, Google, others pledge to watermark AI content for safety, White House says. *Reuters*. https://www.reuters.com/technology/openai-google-others-pledge-watermark-ai-content-safety-white-house-2023-07-21/#:~:text=As%20part%20of%20the%20effort,the%20technology%20has%20been%20used. Accessed 24 July 2023.

Beets, Becca, Todd P. Newman, Emily L. Howell, Luye Bao, and Shiyu Yang. 2023. Surveying public perceptions of artificial intelligence in health care in the United States: Systematic review. *Journal of Medical Internet Research* 25: e40337. https://doi.org/10.2196/40337.

Char, Danton S. 2018. Implementing machine learning in health care: Addressing ethical challenges. *The New England Journal of Medicine* 378: 981–982.

Chossière, Guillaume, Robert Malina, Akshay Ashok, Irene C. Dedoussi, Sebastian D. Eastham, Raymond L. Speth, and Steven R. H. Barrett. 2017. Public health impacts of excess NOx emissions from Volkswagen diesel passenger vehicles in Germany. *Environmental Research Letters* 12 (3): 034014.

Diakopoulos, Nicholas, and Sorelle Friedler. 2016. How to hold algorithms accountable. *MIT Technology Review*. https://www.technologyreview.com/2016/11/17/155957/how-to-hold-algorithms-accountable/. Accessed 24 July 2023.

European Commission. 2021. Proposal for a regulation laying down harmonized rules on artificial intelligence. https://digital-strategy.ec.europa.eu/en/library/proposal-regulation-laying-down-harmonised-rules-artificial-intelligence. Accessed 29 July 2023.

European Parliament. 2023. EU AI Act: first regulation on artificial intelligence. https://www.europarl.europa.eu/news/en/headlines/society/20230601STO93804/eu-ai-act-first-regulation-on-artificial-intelligence. Accessed 13 August 2023.

Executive Office of the President. 2014. Big data: Seizing opportunities, preserving values. https://obamawhitehouse.archives.gov/sites/default/files/docs/big_data_privacy_report_may_1_2014.pdf. Accessed 24 July 2023.

Executive Order 13960. 2020. Promoting the use of trustworthy artificial intelligence in the federal government. *Code of Federal Regulations* 85: 78939–78943.

Feingold, Spencer. 2023. The European Union's artificial intelligence act - explained. *World Economic Forum*. https://www.weforum.org/agenda/2023/06/european-union-ai-act-explained/. Accessed 13 Aug 2023.

Fitzgerald, Madyson. 2023. As employers expand artificial intelligence in hiring, Maryland is one of few states that have rules. *Maryland Matters*. https://www.marylandmatters.org/2023/07/18/as-employers-expand-artificial-intelligence-in-hiring-maryland-is-one-of-few-states-that-have-rules/. Accessed 26 July 2023.

Fonzone, Christopher, and Kate Heinzelman. 2018. Should the government regulate artificial intelligence? It already is. *THE HILL*. http://thehill.com/opinion/technology/375606-should-the-government-regulate-artificial-intelligence-it-already-is. Accessed 10 Aug 2023.

Greenemeier, Larry. 2015. What's behind VW's downfall and secretive emissions deals. *Scientific American*. https://www.scientificamerican.com/article/what-s-behind-vw-s-downfall-and-secretive-emissions-deals/. Accessed 10 Aug 2023.

Guihot, Michael, Anne F. Matthew, and Nicolas P. Suzor. 2017. Nudging robots: Innovative solutions to regulate artificial intelligence. *Vanderbilt Journal of Entertainment and Technology Limited* 20: 385–456.

Hotton, Russell. 2015. Volkswagen: The scandal explained. *BBC*. https://www.bbc.com/news/business-34324772. Accessed 29 July 2023.

Hudson, Laura. 2017. Technology is biased too. How do we fix it? *FiveThirtyEight* https://fivethirtyeight.com/features/technology-is-biased-too-how-do-we-fix-it/. Accessed 29 July 2023.

Isaac, Mike. 2017. How Uber deceives the authorities worldwide. *The New York Times*. https://www.nytimes.com/2017/03/03/technology/uber-greyball-program-evade-authorities.html. Accessed 29 July 2023.

Jillson, Elise. 2021. Aiming for truth, fairness, and equity in your company's use of AI. *U.S. Federal Trade Commission*. https://www.ftc.gov/news-events/blogs/business-blog/2021/04/aiming-truth-fairness-equity-your-companys-use-ai. Accessed 20 April 2021.

Lima, Cristiano, and David DiMolfetta. 2023. Google bucks calls for a new AI regulator. *The Washington Post*. https://www.washingtonpost.com/politics/2023/06/13/google-bucks-calls-new-ai-regulator/. Accessed 24 July 2023.

Lohr, Steven. 2023. A hiring law blazes a path for A.I. regulation. *The New York Times*. https://www.nytimes.com/2023/05/25/technology/ai-hiring-law-new-york.html. Accessed 26 July 2023.

Nader, Karim, Paul Toprac, Suzanne Scott, and Samuel Baker. 2022. Public understanding of artificial intelligence through entertainment media. *AI Society* 2: 1–14. https://doi.org/10.1007/s00146-022-01427-w.

National Conference of State Legislators. 2023. Legislation related to artificial intelligence. https://www.ncsl.org/technology-and-communication/artificial-intelligence-2023-legislation. Accessed 24 June 2023.

New York City. 2019. Automated decision systems task force report. https://www.nyc.gov/assets/adstaskforce/downloads/pdf/ADS-Report-11192019.pdf. Accessed 24 July 2023.

O'Neil, Cathy. 2017. How can we stop algorithms telling lies. *The Guardian*. http://www.cs.otago.ac.nz/staffpriv/ok/lying-algorithms.pdf. Accessed 10 Aug 2023.

OECD.AI. 2021. Database of national AI policies. https://oecd.ai. Accessed 24 July 2023.

Oldenkamp, Rik, Rosalie van Zelm, and Mark A. Huijbregts. 2016. Valuing the human health damage caused by the fraud of Volkswagen. *Environmental Pollution* 212: 121–127.

Reddy, Sandeep, Sonia Allan, Simon Coghlan, and Paul Cooper. 2020. A governance model for AI in health care. *Journal of the American Medical Informatics Association* 27 (3): 491–497.

Richardson, Rashida. 2017. New York City takes on algorithmic discrimination. *ACLU*. https://www.aclu.org/blog/privacy-technology/surveillance-technologies/new-york-city-takes-algorithmic-discrimination. Accessed 29 July 2023.

Satariano, Adam. 2023. Europeans take a major step toward regulating A.I. *The New York Times*. https://www.nytimes.com/2023/06/14/technology/europe-ai-regulation.html#:~:text=A%20draft%20law%20in%20the,harmful%20effects%20of%20artificial%20intelligence.&text=Adam%20Satariano%2C%20a%20technology%20correspondent,covers%20digital%20policy%20in%20Europe. Accessed 13 Aug 2023.

Smith, Andrew. 2020. Using artificial intelligence and algorithms. *U.S. Federal Trade Commission Bureau of Consumer Protection*. https://www.ftc.gov/news-events/blogs/business-blog/2020/04/using-artificial-intelligence-algorithms. Accessed 29 July 2023.

Stanford University. Human Centered Artificial Intelligence. 2021. Summary of AI provisions from the National Defense Authorization Act of 2021. https://hai.stanford.edu/policy/policy-resources/summary-ai-provisions-national-defense-authorization-act-2021. Accessed 29 July 2023.

The White House Office of Science and Technology Policy. 2022. Blueprint for an AI bill of rights. https://www.whitehouse.gov/ostp/ai-bill-of-rights/. Accessed 24 July 2023.

U.S. Environmental Protection Agency. 2015. VW Notice of violation letter. https://www.epa.gov/sites/production/files/2015-10/documents/vw-nov-caa-09-18-15.pdf. Accessed 29 July 2023.

U.S. Environmental Protection Agency. 2020. Volkswagen Clean Air Act civil settlement. https://www.epa.gov/enforcement/volkswagen-clean-air-act-civil-settlement. Accessed 29 July 2023.

U.S. Federal Trade Commission. 2016. Big data. A tool for inclusion or exclusion. https://www.ftc.gov/system/files/documents/reports/big-data-tool-inclusion-or-exclusion-understanding-issues/160106big-data-rpt.pdf. Accessed 12 Aug 2023.

Wyden, Ron. 2019. Wyden, Booker, Clarke introduce bill requiring companies to target bias in corporate algorithms. https://www.wyden.senate.gov/news/press-releases/wyden-booker-clarke-introduce-bill-requiring-companies-to-target-bias-in-corporate-algorithms. Accessed 11 Aug 2023.

Zakrzewski, Cat. 2023. Top tech firms sign White House pledge to identify AI-generated images. *The Washington Post*. https://www.washingtonpost.com/technology/2023/07/21/ai-white-house-pledge-openai-google-meta/. Accessed 22 July 2023.

Index

N. H. Williams, *Artificial Intelligence and Healthcare*, The International Library of Bioethics 107, https://doi.org/10.1007/978-3-031-48262-5